Depression and African American Women

iUniverse, Inc.
New York   Bloomington

Depression and African American Women

iUniverse books may be ordered through booksellers or by contacting:

iUniverse
1663 Liberty Drive
Bloomington, IN 47403
www.iuniverse.com
1-800-Authors (1-800-288-4677)

Contact author:
BRK Healthcare Services Incorporation
Bern29044@Aol.com

Because of the dynamic nature of the Internet, any Web addresses or links contained in this book may have changed since publication and may no longer be valid. The views expressed in this work are solely those of the author and do not necessarily reflect the views of the publisher, and the publisher hereby disclaims any responsibility for them.

ISBN: 978-1-4401-3437-1 (pbk)
ISBN: 978-1-4401-3438-8 (ebk)

Printed in the United States of America

iUniverse rev. date: 11/12/2009

Depression and African American Women

by

Bernice Roberts Kennedy,

RN, PhD, APRN, BC

Perspectives on African American Women and Depression

Black women have waged battles against what has been called the "largest cultural Goliath" in the human history – American dominant, mainstream, hegemonic cultural... even for some of these women, however, reflecting on past experiences at some point becomes necessary for establishing meaning and direction in life (Scott, 199, p.2).

Many Black women in the United States are broken hearted. They walk around in daily life carrying so much hurt, feeling wasted, yet pretending in every area of their life that everything is under control. It hurts to pretend. It hurts to live with lies. The time has come for black women to attend to that hurt..... their (ancestors) healing power can be felt in black women's lives if we dare to look at ourselves, our lives, our experiences and then, without shame, courageously name we see (Hook, 1993, p.29-30).

African American women tend to look at mental health treatment e.g., therapy as a sign of weakness. They present themselves to society as strong, resilient human beings. These characteristics are ingrain in the African American women culture and can be traced back to slavery. Often, African American women pretend she is okay when she is actually suffering inside (Black, 2001).

Often, African American women may be misdiagnosed because they go to health care visits looking well-groomed regardless of feeling depressed or sad. As a result, healthcare professionals often see their appearance as well- groomed, not disheveled during their assessment. When assessing African American females, they often deny feeling depressed because they don't want to be seen as weak or not spiritually strong. In some culture, common phrases of African Americans when referring to their health problems are "I am not going to claim it" or "I 'm bless." (Dr. Bernice Robert Kennedy, 2005)

Cognitive therapy focuses on removing symptoms by identifying and correcting negative behavior. For example, African American women's perception of racism or discrimination may cause " oppressive or negative behaviors " resulting in depressive symptoms. In order to correct these negative behaviors they must change their negative perceptions of their life situations by developing a **sense of empowerment.** *In addition, the stigma associated with seeking mental and emotional health prevents many African women from admitting they are struggling with these issues and identifying alternative solutions. Therapists need to assist African American women in identifying and exploring more positive alternative strategies in problem- solving (Dr. Bernice Roberts Kennedy, 2008).*

For many African American women spirituality is necessary in the concept of healing for depression. Spirituality creates attitudes that embrace hope and empowerment. In a healthy person, spirituality is critical for overall mental health using the network found in the family, neighborhood, church, mosque, temple and community (Mitchell & Herring 2003).

Clinical depression is often a vague disorder for African- American women. It may produce an abundance of "depressions" in the lives of the women who experience its ongoing, relentless symptoms. The old adage of "being sick and tired of being sick and tired" is quite relevant for these women, since they often suffer from persistent, untreated physical and emotional symptoms. If these women consult health professionals, they are frequently told that they are hypertensive, run down, or tense and nervous. They may be prescribed antihypertensives, vitamins, or mood elevating pills; or they may be informed to lose weight, learn to relax, get a change of scenery, or get more exercise. The root of their symptoms frequently is not explored; and these women continue to complain of being tired, weary, empty, lonely and sad. Other women friends and family members may say, "We all feel this way sometimes, it's just the way it is for us Black women" (Warren, 1995. Paragraph, 1).

African American women with depression reported that the language of depression differs from health professionals' nomenclature and the distinctive language of depression. African American women were constructed around the cultural symbol of blues music (Barbee, 1992).

African women experience multiple complex problems because they contended with the stressful issues of gender, race and class in society. They experience stress because of discrimination both within and outside their communities. They may experience racism from other women, as well as men. The combined influence of gender and race broadly impacts the personal development of black women (Brown & McNair 1995).

*African American women express resistance to oppression and racism encountered in the healthcare system through personal relationships with **God and Jesus** and through support and strength found within the church congregation. The women in this study emphasized the influence of a personal belief in Jesus, focusing on **His*** *presence and His power,* on health and resistance to negative experiences within the healthcare system. Overriding all themes was the idea of *Jesus as the true Healer* (M. Abrum, 2004).

Introduction

Depression is gradually increasing in African American women. These women are experiencing role changes and additional life stressors. Depressed African American women may perceive themselves as being devalued by society with fewer support systems to buffer stressful events. Depressive symptoms may develop into clinical depression and further decrease the quality of life for the African American woman. The assumption that all women share similar experiences does not allow for differences to emerge regarding the diagnostic process, measuring tools, and successful treatment strategies for various cultures. Cultural background plays a vital role in how the symptoms of mental illnesses are developed, reported and interpreted, and how women are treated. Also, African American women are more apt to have less access to routine medical care where early diagnosis and interventions can be done, so their mental health problems (e.g., depression, stress, etc.) are often more developed, complicated, and their social supports more depleted when they do access treatment.

The author proposed strategies for improving treatment of African American women with depression and future research needs. The various treatments for depression are discussed to include traditional and alternative/complementary treatments.In addition, culturally competent strategies for improving the treatment of African American women with depression are addressed.

Table of Contents

Chapter 1: Overview of Depression

Depression is a commonly treatable disorder affecting over 19 million American adults every year. Women are approximately (2 times) more likely than men to suffer from Major Depression and Dysthymic Depression Disorders (Research Agenda for Psychosocial and Behavioral Factors in Women's Health, 1996). Depression has been called the most frequent mental health risk for women, especially younger women of childbearing age (Glied & Kofman, 1995). However, depression is gradually increasing in African American women. These women are experiencing role changes and additional stressors. Depressed African American women may perceive themselves as being devalued by society and with fewer support systems to buffer stressful events (Sue & Sue, 2005). Depressive symptoms may develop into clinical depression and further decrease in the quality of life for the African American woman. The assumption that all women share similar experiences does not allow for differences to emerge regarding the diagnostic process, measuring tools, and successful treatment strategies for various cultures (Coridan & O'Connell, 2002).

Black women are at risk than their white counterparts for experiencing stress and negative outcomes in areas such as health, education and psychological well-being. The effects of these oppressive conditions include a serious distorted view of self and others, feeling of hopelessness, and over reliance on maladaptive strategies and isolation (Jone, 2002).

Black women experience multiple problems in their lives because they contend with issues of gender, race and class. They encounter discrimination both within and outside their communities. They may experience racism from other women, as well as men. The combined influenced of gender and race broadly impacts the personal development of black women (Brown & McNair, 1995).

Often, African American women are hindered by fewer years of education, higher rate of unemployment, over-representation in low-status, low-paying jobs, and significant higher rate of poverty than those of white and black men(Miranda, Chung, Green , Krupnick, Siddique, et al., 2003). Within the professional realms, they are under-represented in position of power and generally are denied sufficient access to necessary social and material resources. Black women tend to suffer poorer mental and physical health outcomes than other ethnic groups, regardless of their socioeconomic status (Brown & McNair, 1995; Jones, 2002).

Incidence and Prevalence

Currently, depression affects approximately over 19 million adults every year in the United States. Approximately, 12 million women in the United States experience clinical depression (NMHA, 2004), and the rate among African American women is (50 %) higher than white women (Zauszniewski, et al., 2002).

African Americans account for approximately (25 %) of the mental health needs in this country, though they only make up (11 to 12 %) of the nation population, and only (2 %) of mental health psychiatrists are African Americans (NMHA, 2004). The prevalence of mental disorders is estimated to be higher among African Americans than among White Americans. This disparity is more likely due to economic differences. They are under-represented in some private outpatient population, over-represented in some inpatient population and more likely than White Americans to use the emergency room for mental treatment. African Americans drop out of services at a significantly higher rate than whites and use fewer treatment sessions for mental services (Coridan & O'Connell, 2002). They enter treatment at a later, more advanced stage than White Americans, access at a low rate of community mental health services, and misdiagnosed with a severe mental illness than White Americans (Coridan & O'Connell, 2002).

Clinical research on African American women has been scarce. This scarcity in clinical research is because usually, African American women do not seek treatment for their depression (Coridan & O'Connell, 2002). In addition, they are often misdiagnosed, or may have withdrawn from treatment because their ethnic, cultural, or gender needs are not being met. Often, they do not participate in research studies because they are uncertain as to how research data will be disseminated, or they are afraid that the data will be misinterpreted (Carrington, 2006). African American women, also, are less available to participate in depression research studies resulting in limited empirical data of research findings to improve treatment.

Historical Perspective

At the beginning of the 21st century African American women found themselves achieving new heights and reaching new milestones (Sue & Sue, 2005). Education and hard work enabled them to achieve successful career and respect in the mainstream society. Despite this news, African American women still find themselves lagging behind white women and other women in health and mental health.

Clinical depression is often a vague disorder for African American women. This disorder produces an abundance of depressive symptoms in the lives of women who experience it ongoing, relentless symptoms. African American women often suffer from persistent, untreated physical and emotional symptoms (Warren, 1995). Healthcare providers often tell African American women that they are hypertensive, run down, tense or nervous. Often, healthcare providers prescribe antihypertensive, vitamins, or mood elevating pills for their physical problems. In addition, these healthcare providers may inform them to lose weight, learn to relax, get a change of scenery, or get more exercise. However, the roots of their symptoms are not explored. These women continue to complain of depressive symptoms such as being tire, weary, empty, lonely and sad. Other women, friends, and family members may express to them that they all feel this way and it is indicative of black women (Warren, 1995).

Research indicates that racism has an affect on an individual's mental health (Tinsley-Jones 2003). It was found that racial/ethnic minority groups are at a greater risk of psychiatric issues such as anxiety and depression, which was linked to racism. In addition, it has been reported those African Americans who have been racially discriminated against report lower levels of life satisfaction than African Americans who have not experienced discrimination.

African American women face a multitude of issues and challenges due to discrimination. In the past, African American women struggled with challenges such as discrimination, oppression through slavery, segregation, Jim Crow Laws, an inability to vote, and unequal rights. Although, African American women have made significant strides in today's society, discrimination continues to exist, which leads to further oppression. Other challenges faced by African American women today include the unequal opportunities through education, job opportunities poverty, etc.

Chapter 2: Definition of Depression

Depression is the state wherein an individual experiences a profound sadness. Sadness and loss are universal, but symptoms severe enough to justify a diagnosis of depression are much rare. Depression may range from mild and moderate states to severe state with or without psychotic features. Psychotic feature or psychosis is a symptom of mental illness characterized by a radical change in personality and a distorted diminished sense of objectivity reality. People experiencing psychosis may report hallucinations or delusional beliefs, and may exhibit personality changes and disorganized thinking. Epidemiological studies suggest that (7 to 25 %) of women are likely to become significantly depressed at some time in their lives (Diagnostic and Statistical Manual of Mental Disorders (DSM-IV), (2000).

The DSM-IV makes a fundamental distinction between a mood episode and a depression disorder. A mood episode is the experience of strong emotion of depression, mania, or a mixture of both for a period of at least (2 weeks). The symptoms should be newly present or have clearly worsened over the preepisode state and must be present nearly every day for most of the day for (2 consecutive weeks). A mood disorder is diagnosed based on the pattern of mood episodes.

Clinical Depression is a serious medical illness that is much more than temporary feeling sad or blue (Frisch & Frisch, 2006). It involves disturbances in mood, concentration, sleep, activity, appetite and social behavior. Depression can develop in anyone at any age. Although, depression is treatable, it is frequently a life long condition in which a period of wellness alternate with recurrence of illness.

Signs and Symptoms of Depression

Recognizing the Depression

People who are depressed often have the following characteristics:

- Find that previous enjoyment activities no longer produce the same job

- Loss of interest in friends; isolation from others

- Difficulties concentrating

- A history of significant loss or trauma

- A sense of powerlessness and hopelessness

- Loss of appetite and weight

- Sleep disturbances, particular early morning awaking with inability to fall back asleep

Signs and symptoms of depression consist of psychological and physical signs and symptoms.

Psychological Signs and Symptoms

Psychological sign and symptoms consist of the following:

- Depressed mood (sad)

- Reduction in interest and/or pleasure in activities, including sex

- Feelings of guilt, hopelessness and worthlessness

- Suicidal thoughts (recurrent)

Physical Signs and Symptoms

Physical signs and symptoms are as follows:

- Sleep disturbance (insomnia or hypersomnia)

- Appetite/weight changes

- Attention/concentration difficulties

- Decreased energy or unexplained fatigue

- Psychomotor disturbance (decreased movement; slow thoughts and impaired capacity to work; slowing

and/or agitation of physical movement)

Suicide

Approximately 30,000 people complete the act of suicide each year. Suicide is the eighth leading cause of death in the United States and the third leading killer of young people.   Males commit the majority of complete suicides. In addition, males typically shoot themselves, women attempt suicide (3 times) as often as men, using potentially less lethal means such as medication and wrist cutting. However, one third of women who complete suicide; and over half of those are 15 to 29 years of age use guns (Stuart & Laraia, 2004). Black women have the lowest suicide rates in the United States. However, they have a higher incidence of depression than their white counterpart.

The suicide rate for African American for all age was (5:25 per 100,000) about half the overall United States rate of (10.75 per 100.000). Suicide is the third leading cause of death for African American the ages of 15 and 24 (CDC, 2007). The risk for attempted suicide is highest among 15 and 24 years of age. Younger generations of African Americans are at significant higher risk for suicide attempts (Joe, 2006).

African American beliefs about suicide may affect the suicide rates. Religious communities condemn suicide while secular attitudes regard suicide is an unacceptable behavior in their culture (Early & Akers, 1993).

Black women attempt suicide almost the same rate as white women but have less completion (Goldsmith, 2001). One study found that when compared to white women, black women have greater social support, extend families, more religious view against suicide and stronger mothering philosophies, all of which may act as protective factors (Williams, González, Neighbors, Nesse, Abelson, Sweetman, et al., (2007).

Risk Factors

Approximately (15 %) of severely depressed patients commit suicide. Other complications include martial, parental, and social, and vocational difficulties.

Risk for Suicidal Attempts

- Age less than 30 years

- Threatened loss of intimate relationship

- Live alone

- Current psychosocial stressors (e.g., loss of job)

- Substance abuse

- Personality disorders (e.g., Borderline Personality

Disorder)

Risk Factors for Complete Suicide

- Severe clinical depression, especially with psychosis

- Past history of suicidal attempts

- Current active suicidal ideation or plan

- Divorced or more active or chronic medical illnesses

- Feeling of hopelessness

- Panic disorder

- Severe anxiety, especially with mixed depression

Risk Factors for African Americans

The risk factors for suicide among African Americans are as follows:

- Being under age 35

- Residing in southern and northeastern states

- Using cocaine

- Having a firearm in the home

- Threatening others with violence (Willis, Coombs, Drentea, & Cockerham, 2003).

Chapter 3: Types of Depression

The 3 primary   types of depressive disorders are Major Depression Disorder, Dysthymic Disorder and Manic Depression or Bipolar   Depression Disorder. The medical diagnosis of Major Depression Disorder (also called Unipolar Disorder) is a loss of interest in life. A person experiences a depressed mood from mild to severe, with the severe phase lasting (2 weeks). It is twice as common in females than in males. Some people with Major Depression Disorder may experience delusions and hallucinations. When this occurs, it is referred to as severe depression with psychotic features (e.g., hallucinations, delusions, disorganized or illogical thinking). Dysthymic Disorder is a chronic disorder in which periods of depressed moods are interspersed with normal moods. People with Dysthymic Disorder are at high risks of developing a superimposed   major depressive episode.

Other types of depression and mood disorders common in women are Seasonal Affective Disorder (SAD), Minor Depression Disorder, Postpartum Depression Disorder, Premenstrual Dysphoric Disorder, and Major Depression Disorder or Bipolar Disorders. They will be discussed in this section.

The common types of depression and mood disorders in women are as follows:

- Major Depression Disorder

- Minor Depression Disorder

- Manic Depression or Bipolar Disorder

- Dysthymic Depression Disorder

- Seasonal Affective Disorder

- Perinatal Depression/Postpartum Blues

- Postpartum Depression

- Premenstrual Dysphoric Disorder (PMDD)

- Perimenopause/Menopause Depression

Major Depressive Disorder

A person experiencing a depressive episode may express feelings of sadness and hopelessness or may express the sense of feeling empty or having no feelings (Frisch & Frisch, 2006). Some persons express somatic symptoms such as bodily aches and pains rather than sadness. Major Depression Disorder begins at any age (Warren, 1995). However, it usually begins in mid-twenties and thirties with the symptoms developing over days to weeks at a time.

The DSM-IV requires the presence of at least one episode to qualify as a Major Depressive Disorder.

- This episode must last at least (2 weeks) and must:

1. Represent a change from previous functioning

2. Cause some impairment in the person's social or occupational functioning

- The individual must also experience (at least 4) addition symptoms of the following:

1. Change in appetite or weight

2. Sleep disturbance (usually trouble staying asleep)

3. Fatigue or loss of energy

4. Feeling of worthlessness or guilt

5. Difficulty concentrating, thinking, or making a decision

6. Recurrent thought of death or suicide

Minor Depressive Disorder

An additional (10 %) of persons may suffer less severe symptoms that may interfere with their functioning but may not qualify for a diagnosis of Major Depressive Disorder. The diagnosis of Minor Depressive Disorder has been proposed for these individuals but has not yet been validated with The American Psychiatric Association Diagnostic Statistical Manual of Mental Disorders (DSM-IV).

Dysthymic Depression Disorder

Dysthymic Depression Disorder differs from Major Depression Disorder in that it is a chronic, low-level depression. Major Depressive Disorder is a discrete episode of depression. Persons with Dysthymic Depression Disorder feel depressed nearly all the time. Dysthymic Depression Disorder includes a depressed mood for most of the day, nearly every day, for at least (2 years). Women have a higher incidence of Dysthymic Depression Disorder than men.

A person with Dysthymic Depression Disorder must also have (at least 2) of the following symptoms:

1. Appetite disturbance

2. Sleep disturbance

3. Fatigue

4. Low self- esteem

5. Poor concentration or difficulty making decisions, and feelings of hopelessness

After (2 years) of Dysthymia, a person may be diagnosed with Major Depression Disorder superimposed on Dysthymia if symptoms increase in severity. The Dysthymic Depression Disorder is not due to the effects of a substance or medical condition. Psychotic features (e.g., hallucinations, delusions, disorganized or illogical thinking) are usually not present in this disorder.

Manic Depression Disorder/ Bipolar Disorder

Manic Depression Disorder is also called **Bipolar Disorder**. This type of depression is not nearly as common as other forms of depression. It involves disruptive cycles of depressive symptoms that alternate with euphoria, irritable excitement, or mania. In addition to severe depression, manic episodes may occur (Frisch & Frisch, 2006). These manic episodes like depression, can vary in intensity and accompanying levels of anxiety from moderate manic states to severe and panic states with psychotic features (e.g., hallucinations, delusions, disorganized or illogical thinking). Mania is characterized by elevated, expansive, or irritable mood. Hypomania is a clinical symptoms similar to but not as severe as mania   (Frisch & Frisch, 2006). In the DSM-IV, the Major Affective Disorders are separated into two groups- Bipolar and Depressive Disorder based on whether manic and depressive episodes are involved longitudinally. In this classification, Major Depressive Disorder may involved a single episode or a recurrent depressive illness but without manic episodes. It is estimated that 2 million Americans have Bipolar Disorders.

The risk factors are being female and having a family history of Bipolar Disorder (Stuart & Laraia, 2004).

Seasonal Affective Disorder (SAD)

Seasonal Affective Disorder (SAD) is depression that comes with shortened daylight in winter and fall and disappears during the spring and summer (Frisch & Frisch, 2006; Stuart & Laraia, 2004). Women are diagnosed with SAD more often than men. The majority of SAD sufferers are women with a family history of mood disorders. Unlike Major Depression Disorder in which children and adults differ, children and adults with SAD exhibit the same symptoms. It is characterized by hypersomnia, lethargy and fatigue, increased irritability, increased appetite with carbohydrate craving, and often weight gain (NIMH, 2008). These symptoms seen more frequently in SAD compared to other mood disorders. However, in other mood disorders the common symptoms are increased appetite, carbohydrate craving and weight gain. SAD is believed to be related to abnormal melatonin metabolism. It has been noted that (2 to 3 times) as many people are troubled by winter reoccurrence of seasonal mood symptoms that exhibit severe enough to merit clinical diagnosis (Stuart & Laraia, 2004). Persons with SAD often develop depression during **October and November** and find it remitting in **March and April.**

Perinatal Depression

Perinatal depression occurs during pregnancy or within a year after delivery (NIMH, 2008). The exact number of women with depression during this time is unknown. Often, the depression is not recognized or treated, because some normal pregnancy changes cause similar symptoms and are happening at the same time. Tiredness, problems sleeping, stronger emotional reactions, and changes in body weight may occur during pregnancy and after pregnancy (NIMH, 2008). But these symptoms may also be signs of depression. The reasons women get depressed are contributed to hormone changes or a stressful life event, such as a death in the family, which can cause chemical changes in the brain that lead to depression. Depression is also an illness that runs in some families. Other times, it's not clear what causes depression.

During pregnancy, these factors may increase a woman's chance of depression:

- History of depression or substance abuse

- Family history of mental illness

- Little support from family and friends

- Anxiety about the fetus

- Problems with previous pregnancy or birth

- Marital or financial problems

- Young age (of mother)

After pregnancy, hormonal changes in a woman's body may trigger symptoms of depression. During pregnancy, the amount of 2 female hormones, estrogen and progesterone, in a woman's body increases greatly. In the first 24 hours after childbirth, the amount of these hormones rapidly drops back down to their normal nonpregnant levels. Researchers think the fast change in hormone levels may lead to depression, just as smaller changes in hormones can affect a woman's mood before she gets her menstrual period (NMHA, 2004).

Postpartum Depression/Postpartum Blues

Mood disorders in women after delivering a baby are fairly common. Symptoms can be described along a continuum from postpartum blues to postpartum depression to the rare form of postpartum psychosis (e.g., hallucinations, delusions, disorganized or illogical thinking etc.) (NIMH, 2008).

Postpartum blues begins within the first days of postpartum and last a few days to (2 weeks) with symptoms disappearing spontaneously. The mood with symptoms may disappear spontaneously. The mood may be unstable, accompanied by sadness, weepiness, irritability, anxiety and fatigue (NIMH, 2008). Approximately, (80 %) of new mothers may experience these symptoms caused by hormonal fluctuations. Most of these women had no previous emotional problems (Weinberg, Posener, DeBattista, Kalehzan, Rothschild, & Shear, 2001).

Postpartum depression is estimated to occur in (10 to 16 %) of new mothers; often beginning within (3 months) of delivery but occur at any time during the first year after having a child. Women with this diagnosis experience the following symptoms:

- Insomnia (i.e., difficulties sleeping)

- Loss of energy

- Inability to concentrate

- Anxiety

- Mood swings

- Periods of crying

- Feelings of despair (ruminates over perceived inadequacies as a mother)

If the depression is untreated, it will affect the ability to parent and to cope with stressful situations. These symptoms must be more intense and longer lasting than (2 weeks) to qualify as postpartum depression. Contributing factors are hormonal changes, family history of depression, feeling overwhelmed by parenting tasks, changes in family dynamics and inadequate support. Women who develop postpartum depression are at an increased risk for depression after subsequent pregnancies (Bloch, Schmidt, Danaceau, Murphy, Nieman, & Rubinow, 2000).

One woman in a thousand experiences a postpartum psychosis (e.g., hallucinations, delusions, disorganized or illogical thinking), which is a medical emergency. The incidence relapse for women who have a diagnose of Bipolar Disorder is (25 to 40 %) during postpartum or 260 women per 1000 deliveries. The symptoms usually occur between the first (2 to 3 weeks) after delivery but may occur as early as 48 hours postpartum. Symptoms develop rapidly and include the following:

- Insomnia (e.g., difficulties sleeping)

- Hallucinations

- Agitation

- Bizarre feelings or behaviors

The mother may have an inordinate concern with the baby's health, particular about lack of love, and delusions (e.g. false beliefs) about the infant being dead. The mother may deny having given birth or hallucinates (e.g., hears voices that command her to hurt the baby). In extreme cases, the mother may even kill the child and/or herself (Jones & Craddock, 2001).

Between (30 to 75%) of women experience mild postpartum "blues" lasting (4 to 10 days). This Postpartum depression is characterized by labile mood, tearfulness, irritability, anxiety, and sleep and appetite disturbances. Patient education and reassurance are generally adequate treatment measures. If physical symptoms and depressed mood persist for (2 weeks), patients should be evaluated for postpartum, Major Depression Disorder, particularly if they have a history of depression (Bhatia & Bhatia, 1999).

Important strategies for helping postpartum mothers are as follows:

- Get as much sleep as possible (e.g., nap when the baby nap)

- Request assistance with household chores and breast feedings

- Request friend, family member, or professional support person to help in the home for part of the day

- Express feelings with husband, partner, family and friends

- Avoid spending too much time alone (e.g., leave the house, run an errand or take a short walk)

- Spend quality time with your husband or partner

- Talk with other mothers, to learn from their experiences

- Join a support group for women with depression

Avoid major   life changes during pregnancy e.g. changes can cause unneeded stress (Roco, 2005)

Premenstrual Dysphoric Disorder (PMDD)

The DSM-IV classifies Premenstrual Dysphoric Disorder (PMDD) under research diagnostic criteria as depression not otherwise specified. Mood and anxiety symptoms can occur only during the premenstrual period, or preexisting symptoms can become worse at this time.

PMDD is identified by somatic and emotional symptoms, which may begin at the luteal onset and end, resolved at the follicular phase. A history of PMDD is a risk factor for Major Depressive Disorder.

Healthcare providers need to identify and treat symptoms that have a significant effect on patients. Dismissing the symptoms as just   premenstrual changes deprives women of potentially beneficial of treatment (DSM-IV, 2000).

PMDD is a severely distressing and debilitating and condition that requires treatment. Between (3% to 8%) of women meet the diagnostic criteria for this disorder, which is presented with symptoms of depression and anxiety as well as cognitive and physical symptoms. The diagnosis of PMDD requires the presence of (5 of 11 symptoms), with at least (1 of the first 4 symptoms) experienced during the last week of the luteal phase as indicated:

1. Depressive Symptoms

- Markedly depressed mood, feelings of hopelessness, self depreciation

- Suddenly feeling sad or tearful, with increased sensitivity to personal rejection

- Decrease interest in activity

- Lethargy, fatigue, marked lack of energy

- Marked changes in appetite and craving for certain foods

- Insomnia or hypersomnia (sleeping to much)

2. Anxiety Symptoms

- Marked anxiety, tension, feelings of being "keyed up" or on "edge"

- Feeling overwhelmed or out of control

3. Cognitive Symptoms

- Subjective sense of having difficulties concentrating

4. Physical Symptoms

- Breast tenderness or swelling, headaches, joint pain, weight gain, bloated feeling (DSM-IV, 2000).

The remission of symptoms must occur within a few days of the onset of menstruation. The symptoms should not represent the exacerbation of preexisting anxiety, depression or personality disorders. PMDD has a greater risk of future depression during pregnancy, the postpartum period and the perimenopausal period suggesting a biochemical relationship between depression and the disorder. Both nonpharmacologic and pharmacologic measures have been implemented in the treatment of PMDD (Bhatia & Bhatia, 1999).

Factors such as a history of depression or PMDD, younger age, limited social support, living alone, greater number of children, marital conflict and ambivalence about pregnancy increase the risk of depression during pregnancy and the postpartum period. A history of depression during the antenatal phase remains one of the strongest predictors of future depression during pregnancy and the puerperium (Bhatia & Bhatia, 1999).

It is believed that postpartum depression can affect the infant by causing delays in language development, problems with emotional bonding to others, behavioral problems, lower activity levels, sleep problems and distress (NIMH, 2008). It is important for father or another caregiver to assist in meeting the needs of the baby and other children in the family while mom is depressed (NIMH, 2008)

Perimenopause/Menopause Depression

Perimenopause or menopause transition begins months or years before the menopause and marked by hormonal changes. The women experience symptoms such as hot flashes, deep disruptions, mood disorders and vaginal changes . Perimenopause begin in women approximately between the ages of 45.5 and 45.7 in the United States lasting 4 years until menopause (Wise, Krieger, Zierier, & Harlow, 2002).

The association of depression with menopause remains a somewhat controversial topic . Early research suggested that menopause problems increased the risk for depression and this mood disorder is referred to as involutional melancholia. Decreasing levels of estrogen during the perimenopausal and menopause year complicate the study of depression in older women. There is an overlap of symptoms between menopause and depression causing diagnoses to be difficulty among healthcare professionals. Reduction in estrogen is known to initiate mood frustrations, diminish sexual drive, and these signs and symptoms are suggestive of peripheral neuropathy in some women (Alexander, 2007). In addition, symptoms of low energy, poor concentration, and sleep disturbances, weight changes and low libido fit the profile in both conditions. A biochemical relationship exists between depression and menopause (Alexander, 2007; Griffith & Lustman, 1997).

Recent studies by SWAN reports a significantly increase of depression in women entering the menopause. Women had the highest risk of depression in the early post-menopausal stage or in women using hormonal therapy compared to women in premenopausal women. In addition, women were likely to have clinical depression in the late perimenopausal stage compared to the early stage. The use of hormonal therapy was a contributing factor (Santoro & Green, 2009). Research found increase premature and early menopause in African American and Hispanic women. However, Japanese American women report the least (Santoro & Green, 2009).

African American women report more symptoms of hot flashes than non-Hispanic Caucasian; however, they are more likely to be overweight and obese, thus, increasing the risk for hot flashes (Santoro & Green, 2009). Stressful lifestyle events were the stronger predictor of depression in the perimenopausal and menopause women. Other predictors of depression were low support and frequent vasomotor symptom (e.g., hot flashes). Women with hot flashes have a higher rate of depression . Other risk factors as reported by other studies include smoking, a history of depression, health related issues, social support and daily stressors (Alexander, 2007). Psychosocial factors have been related to depression in women with menopause such as poor lifestyle (e.g., smoking, little exercise, financial difficulties, lower educational levels, health problems, lack of partners and single parenting (Alexander, 2007).

Both nonpharmacologic and pharmacologic measures have been employed in the treatment of depression in menopause (Bhatia & Bhatia, 1999).   Estrogen replacement therapy is useful in treating the minor depressive symptoms of menopausal women with non-clinical depression. Antidepressant Therapy is initiated if mood symptoms become more severe and enduring and progress to full-blown depression (Cohen, Soares, & Joffe, 2005; Griffith & Lustman, 1997).

Chapter 4: Factors Affecting Depression in African American Women

It has been difficult to treat mental health problems in African American women (Coridan & O'Connell, 2002). African American women tend to minimize the serious nature of their problems (Mitchell & Herring, 2003). Many believe their problem is just the blues and they are not proactive in changing their condition (Barbee, 1992). Historically, African American placed a stigma on mental health problems as a sign of weakness not an illness. In African American culture, the woman often feels they can take care of the problem on their own (Mitchell & Herring, 2003).

Biopsychosocial-Spiritual factors affect depression and health outcomes of African Americans. There are some experiences similar in this group, however, individual makeup needs to be considered. This section includes factors affecting depression in African American women. Sociodemographic factors affecting depression in African American women are as follows: (a) environmental factors, (b) socioeconomic factors (SES), (c) health factors, and (d) cultural factors. Psychosocial factors influencing positive or negative outcomes of African American women with depression are (a) stress factors, (b) coping factors and (c) social support factors *Refer to Table 1: Conceptual Model of Strategies for Improving Depression in African American Women, page, 59).*

Sociodemographic Factors

Environmental Factors

Overall, environmental factors have contributed to the mental health problems (e.g. depression, stress, etc.) of African American women, such as racism in society (Sigelman & Welch 1991; Rouse 2001). African American women live in a majority-dominated society that frequently devalues their ethnicity, culture and gender (McGrath, Strickland, & Russo, 1990). They may perceive factors in the environment, such as sub-standard housing, living in areas of health hazards (e.g., landfills; contaminated water supplies, etc.), fewer years of education, lack of skilled labor and managerial jobs, and over representation in low paying jobs, living in drug infested and violence communities and other ethnic discrimination as racism which may cause depression, stress, etc. (Kennedy, 2009; LaVeist, 2000).

In addition, their stressful living conditions such as poverty, discrimination, racism, abuse and rejection from American society may contribute to their thoughts of suicide (Black, 2003). The lifestyles of African American women have been influenced by poverty and prior injustices, which have molded their worldview of health and illness.

Socioeconomic Factors

African American women are more likely than Caucasian women to share a high level of socioeconomic risk factors for depression. Some socioeconomic factors that contribute to depression are as follows: (a) racial/ ethnic discrimination, (b) lower education and income level, (c) segregation into low status, (d) high job stress, (e) unemployment, (f) poor health, (g) large family sizes, (h) marital dissolution, (i) single parenthood, (j) and low self-esteem (Belle & Doucet, 2003; Jesse, Walcott-Quigg, & Swanson, 2005, Martin, 2003; McGrath et al., 1990). They find themselves at the lower spectrum of the political and economic continuum. African American women are involved in multiple roles in their struggler to survive economically, and advance their roles and families through the mainstream of society. Often, these socioeconomic factors intensify the stress in their lives, which erodes their self- esteem and social systems and health (Warren 1995). Regardless of their socioeconomic status, African American women tend to suffer poorer mental and physical health outcomes than other ethnic groups (Brown & McNair, 1995).

Black women's mental health is affected by their double minority status of being black and female in America (Warren, 1995). The exact incidences of depression in black women are unclear because of the controversy regarding misdiagnosis and lack of clinical research. Black women report depression more often than black men. However, little is known about the sociodemographic indicators of risk and depressive symptoms (Barbee, 1992; Jones-Webb & Snowden, 1993).

African Americans primary roots have originated from West Africa which have reflected some of their cultural traditional and patterns common to West Africans such as a strong family network and belief in spirituality (Kennedy, Mattis, & Woods, 2007; Stewart, 2004; Tillman, 2002). They perceive health as a dynamic process of the mind, body, and spirit (Amankwaa 2003; Mitchell & Herrings 2003). African Americans are represented in every socioeconomic group but the great majority live in poverty and they remain disproportionately poor (Mitchell & Herrings, 2003). In the United States, they have a diverse culture perspective deriving from geographic origins, religion, and different levels of acculturation, intermarriage and socioeconomic status (LaVeist, 2000).

Health Factors

Research studies have reported an association with medical problems and depression (NIMH, 2008; NMHA, 2004). Approximately, one third of patients with medical conditions in hospitals report symptoms of mild or moderate symptoms of depression and up to one fourth may have a depressive illness (NIMH, 2008; NMHA, 2004). African American women have numerous medical problems, in addition to a higher incidence of depression (Bender, 2005). Common health problems in African American women associated with depression are cardiovascular, stroke, diabetes, cancer and obesity (Bender, 2005; Martin, 2008; NIMH, 2008). Also, depression coexist with medical conditions such are heart disease, stroke, cancer, HIV/AIDS, diabetes, Parkinson's disease, thyroid problems and multiple sclerosis. In addition, depression coexisting with these medical conditions may make these conditions worse (NIMH, 2008) . The intensity and frequency of depression are highest in the more severely ill clients. Research has revealed a high incidence of depression among hospitalized patients with serious medical conditions. Often, these depressive symptoms are unrecognized and thus are untreated by healthcare professionals (NMHA, 2004). Research has shown that persons having depression and a serious medical conditions tend to have more severe symptoms of both. These coexisting illnesses impact on positive outcomes such as patients adapting to their medical conditions and increase in medical cost (NIMH, 2008).

Depression often coexist with other mental health disorders such as eating disorders e.g., Anorexia Nevosa, Bulimia Nervosa. Also, anxiety disorders such as Post-traumatic Stress Disorder (PTSD), Obsessive-Compulsive Disorder, Panic Disorder, social phobia and generalized anxieties are associated with depression in women. Women are more prone than men to have coexisting anxiety disorders. For example, women with PTSD may have experience a traumatic event such a sexual abuse, rape, etc. Men are more apt to have more alcohol and substance abuse or dependence coexisting with depression (NIMH, 2008).

African American women often eat or drink heavily to overcome their emotions (Black, 2003). Obesity may contribute to the developing of depression in African American women. There is a negative association between obesity and mental well- being (Bender, 2005). In addition, minority women are more likely to have depression and PTSD. A strong link exists between PTSD, misuse and use of abuse of drugs alcohol and other drugs to include tobacco (Coridan & O'Connell, 2002).

Women who smoke experience adverse reproductive outcomes. High rates of occurrence exist between depression and disorders such as anxiety, substance addiction/abuse (Breslau, Kilbey, & Adreski, 1993).

Smoking cessation may be complicated by factors such as weight gain, tension, anxiety, and irritability (Coridan & O'Connell, 2002).

The treatment of African American women by health care providers are based on their interpretation of cultural perspective in the way African Americans report symptoms of mental illness and substance abuse/ addictions. African American women are more apt to have less access to routine medical care where early diagnosis and interventions can be done. So their mental health problems are often more developed and complicated, and their social supports more depleted when they to access treatment (Coridan & O'Connell, 2002).

Depression has often been misdiagnosed in communities of color because of cultural barriers such as language, trust, and values in the relationship between doctor and patient, and reliance on the support of family and the religious community rather than mental health professionals during periods of emotional distress (Black, 2001; Coridan & O'Connell, 2002). Many individuals in minority culture "mask" depressive symptoms with other medical conditions, such as, somatic complaints, substance abuse/addiction and other psychiatric illnesses (Stock, 2005).

Culture Factors/Spiritual Factors

Culture plays an important role in the development of depression in African American women (Amankwaa, 2003). Also, there is a stigma associated with seeking mental and emotional health that prevents many African American women from admitting they are struggling with mental health issues (Black, 2001). Historically, mental health has been viewed as demonic or evil in the African American community (Amankwaa, 2003). Typically, African Americans suffering from mental health problems may not seek or access the mental health system. In some cultures, root doctors were a preferred treatment or religious leaders for spiritual interventions. When African American women enter the health care system, their cultural presentation of self and reporting information to health care providers of different races may be misinterpreted (Barbee, 1992). The misinterpretation of information provided may lead to inappropriate diagnosis and treatment interventions.

Often, African Americans will seek treatment from the community or a religious leader rather than a mental health professional (Coridan & O'Connell 2002). Traditionally, mental health services have not been sensitive to ethnic differences in the ways their clients e.g., African Americans recognize, define, and express symptoms of emotional distress (Mills , 2000).

African American women tend to look at mental health treatment (e.g., therapy as a sign of weakness). They present themselves to society as strong, resilient individuals. These characteristics are ingrain in the

African American women culture and can be traced back to slavery. Often, African American women pretend she is okay when she is actually suffering inside (Black, 2003).

In some cultures, African American women feel they need to pray and keep the problems within the black community. They feel that they are not being the strong black women if they admit having a problem and telling a stranger about their problems (Black, 2003).

African Americans often mistrust the mental health professionals based on history due to higher than average institutionalization of African Americans with mental illness (Coridan & O'Connell, 2002). There is a stigma associated with seeking mental and emotional health that prevents many blacks women from admitting they are struggling with issues. Less than (10 %) of African Americans suffering from depression seek help. Cultural barriers, including the presentation of symptoms may influence language and behavior mannerisms (Barrow, 2003). African American population often rely on the support of family and religious community, rather than mental health professionals, during a period of emotional distress. In addition, African American women may mask symptoms of depression by other medical conditions, somatic complaints, substance use and other psychiatric illness (Barrow, 2003; Coridan & O'Connell, 2002).

In a study of African American women with depression, Barbee reported that the language of depression differed from health professionals' nomenclature and the distinctive language of depression. African American women were constructed around the cultural symbol of blues music. African American world-views are concerned with family and group survival in American society. This worldview emphasizes one's spirituality, interdependence within element of the universe with less emphasis place on material goods. This worldview may have some bearing on African American women's ways of experiencing depression (Amankwaa, 2003).

Treatment of African American women may be based on presentation of illness, interpretation of symptoms of health care providers. When African American women enter the health care system, their cultural presentation of self and reporting information to health care providers of different races may be misinterpreted (Barbee, 1992). The misinterpretation of information provided may lead to inappropriate diagnosis, and treatment interventions.

Psychosocial Factors

Stress Factors

Various psychological, individual behavior, and cultural factors may influence how individuals perceive and response to environmental stimuli. These factors may play a major role in the the presentation or treatment of almost every general medical conditon (e.g., depression, physical or other mental health problems). Stress has been found to be associated with higher rates of somatic and psychiatric illnesses (Cohen & Williamson 1991).

Racism may be preceived as a stressor in the environment of African American women (LaVeist, 2000). African American women are more at risk for depression than their white counterparts for experiencing stress and negative outcomes in areas such as health. The effects of this oppression may include a seriously distorted view of self and others, feelings of hopelessness, and over reliance on maladaptive strategies to include isolation (Jones, 2002). African women experience multiple complex problems because they contended with the stressful issues of gender, race and class in society. They experience stress because of discrimination both within and outside the communities. They may experience racism from other women, as well as men. The combined influence of gender and race broadly impacts the personal development of black women (Brown & McNair 1995).

Coping Factors

Coping is defined as those abilities that enable an individual to buffer the negative effects of stress or psychosocial vulnerability. General coping responses refer to strategies that are usually used to deal with stressful events (Folkman & Lazarus, 1980). Coping mechanisms operate by either eliminating the source of the stress (e.g., solving a pressuring problem) or decreasing the unpleasant effect of stress (e.g., talking about feelings with a friend, family, spiritual leader, overeating, etc.

Depression is a stigma in the African American community. African American women often feel guilty and don't want their families to see them as weak. Some of the symptoms of depression such as not eating, not sleeping and lack of motivation are more reasons for the major population to confirm the stereotype that African Americans are lazy and shiftless, so African Americans often deny they suffer from depression (Black, 2003).

Numerous psychological responses may follow perceptions of racism such as depression, stress, fears, distrust, paranoia, anger, etc. (Clark, Anderson, Clark, & Williams, 1999). Some African American women may grow up in a household with high levels of depression and inadequate coping mechanisms. However, the coping mechanisms of African American women are based on cultural practices. In a survey by NMHA on attitudes about depression, about (63 %) of African Americans believe that depression is a personal weakness, compared to the overall average of (54 %). Only, (31 %) of African Americans said they considered depression a health problem. Approximately, (30 %) of African Americans said they could handle depressive feelings on their own. The survey concluded that only (25 %) of African Americans recognized that a change in eating and sleeping patterns is a sign of depression. Only one-third of African Americans said that they would take medication for depression, if prescribed by a doctor, compared to (69 %) of the general population. Almost two-thirds, of respondents said they believe prayer and faith alone will successfully treat depression "almost all of the time" or "some of the time" (NMHA, 2000).

Social Support Factors

It is the amount of psychosocial assistance that a person perceives is readily available from the people with whom he/she has regular contact (family, friends, colleagues, spiritual leaders etc.). High levels of social support generally are associated with postive health outcomes and have been found to protect individuals from the negative effects of stress (a buffering effect) (Cohen & Wills 1985).

Research findings have reported that the psychological well-being of African Americans is enhanced by a satisifactory marriage and threatened by an unsatisfactory marriage. African Americans experience greater strains and more unhappy marriages than White Americans (Mitchell & Herring, 2003). Lower levels of spousal support and financial satisfaction among African Americans make a significant contribution to these racial differences. Among African Americans who were legally married or in long-term common-law marriages, maritial strain is associated with higher levels of depression (Keith & Norword, 1997). Other social support systems for the African American females are family, and religious leaders. Also, African American women seek healing through other women with similar experience (Mitchell & Herring, 2003).

African American women tend to rely on supports of others than rely on the mental health services. The community, family, and the religious community are support systems African women rely on during periods of emotional distress. Black women seek mental health care less than white women (Coridan & O'Connell, 2002).

Chapter 5: Traditional Treatment of Depression

Overview of Treatment

Current treatments for depression include psycho-therapy, somatic or physical therapies and medications (Frisch & Frisch, 2006). African American women need to understand that depression is not a weakness, but an illness often resulting from a combination of causes (Warren, 1995). Antidepressants are useful for treat-ing neurochemical imbalances or physical disorders. Psychotherapy is effective for depression. However, certain surgeries or certain conditions e.g., heart, dia-betes, hormonal, blood pressure, or kidney medications actually induce depression (Warren, 1995). African American women may require being more sensitivity to certain antidepressants requiring smaller dosages. (McGrath et al., 1990). However, it is useful for women during pregnancy or trying to conceive to avoid possible side effects on the developing fetus that may result from the use of some medications.

The focus of individual or group psychotherapy is to enhance their self-esteem, and develop alternative strategies in order to handle their stress and conflicting roles appropriately (Warren, 1995). African American women should learn relaxation techniques, and develop alternative coping and crisis strategies. Group sessions may be more supportive for some women and may facilitate the development of wider selections of life-style choice and changes. Self-help groups may provide social support for depressed African American women to enhance the work accomplished in therapeutic set-tings. African American women need to monitor their on-going emotional and physical health as they progress in life (Warren, 1995).

Psychotherapy

Psychotherapies include are as follows:

- Brief dynamic therapy- focuses on core conflicts that derive from personality and living situations.

- Marital therapy- attempts to resolve problem that occur with a marriage.

- Cognitive therapy- focuses on removing symptoms by identifying and correcting perceptual bias in client's thinking and correcting unrecognized assumptions.

- Psychotherapy alone helps some depressed persons, especially those with mild to moderate symptoms (Frisch & Frisch, 2006). Studies have reported that psychotherapy has fairly consistent benefit for depression. Depression can be treated successfully by antidepressant medications in (65 %) of cases. Success rate of treatment increases to (85 %) when alternative or adjunctive medications are used or psychotherapy is combined with medications (Young, Klap, Sherbourne, & Well, 2000).

Psychotherapy and drug treatment work much better for low-income young minority women than referrals to community health services. Medications have been effective for poor and minority women if they are given support to overcome barriers to care. When used properly, medications appear to give better result than psychotherapies (Young, et al., 2000). However, effective treatment for minority women had been questioned because depression treatment guidelines are based largely on white or college-educated patients. This left a gap in the knowledge of treating low-income and minority women (Leven, 2003).

Antidepressant Medications

There is no clear evidence of gender differences in the effectiveness of antidepressants medications. However, women typically experience more adverse effects than men.   Selective Serotonin Uptake Inhibitors (SSRI)-(Prozac, Zoloft, Paxil, Luvox) have fewer side effects. Some doctors suggested increasing dose of antidepressant drugs premenstrually, as the menstrual cycle may alter drug-absorption rates (Blumenthal & Endicott, 1996).

Because of the potential risk of the developing fetus or newborn, the cost and benefits of the use of antidepressants must be weight carefully for women who are pregnant, breast-feeding, or trying to conceive. Studies have not shown any significant increase in birth defects in children of women using Tricyclic antidepressants (e.g., Anafranil, Elavil, Pamelar) or SSRI during pregnancy (Blumenthal & Endicott, 1996). However, MAOIs (e.g., Nardil, Parnate) may adversely affect the developing fetus and lead to complications during delivery. Lithium (commonly prescribed for Bipolar Disorder) has been linked to increase birth defects. However, many healthy babies have been born to mothers using this medication (Blumenthal & Endicott, 1996).

The lowest effective dose of medication should be given. Also, the antidepressants with the least sedation and anticholinergic potency (e.g., rapid heartbeat, high blood pressure, slow digestion, dry mouth, constipation, and urinary retention) are used because of possible adverse effects on the newborn. In clients with severe depression, doctors must weight the risks and benefits in both the mother and the infant of using medications as compared to not administering drug therapy (Blumenthal & Endicott, 1996).

Combination of Psychosocial and Pharmacological Interventions

Psychosocial and pharmacologic treatments may be considered (Pajer, 1995). Psychosocial therapies should address issues that particularly affect women, such as competing roles and conflicts. Commonly used treatments include psychotherapy to correct interpersonal conflicts and to help women develop interpersonal skills; cognitive-behavioral therapy to correct negative thinking and associated behavior; and couples therapy to reduce marital conflicts. In patients with mild to moderate depression, psychosocial therapies may be used alone for a limited period, or they may be used in conjunction with antidepressant medication (McGrath, 1990).

Physical Therapies

Common physical therapies are Electroconvulsive Therapy and Light Therapy.

Electroconvulsive Therapy (ECT)

- Electroconvulsive Therapy is a procedure in which clients are treated with pulses of electrical energy sufficient to cause a brief convulsion or seizure.

- Effects of ECT. ECT is utilized in depression because multiple studies have shown it to be highly effective in helping severe depression resistant to other treatments.

Many studies of ECT and depression produce response rate as high as (90 %). In comparison to medication, ECT has been clearly shown to be the superior treatment.

Light Therapy

Light Therapy is a new form of treatment, the indications for which have yet to be completely established. When used for SAD, Light Therapy relieves symptoms in (e.g., 75 %) of persons.

Types of Antidepressant Medications

There are 3 categories of Antidepressant medications. (a) Tricyclic (TCAs), (b) Selective Serotonin Reuptake Inhibitors (SSRIs), and (c) Monoamine Oxidase Inhibitors (MAOIs).

Tricyclics (TCAs) and Related Antidepressants

- Imipramine (Trofanil) was the first antidepressant medication use to treat depression.

- TCAs block monoamine (norepinephrine and serontonin) uptake, thus intensifying the effect of the norephrinephrine and serotonin.

- TCAs can elevate mood, increase activity and alertness, decrease a client's preoccupation with morbidity, improve appetite and regulate sleep pattern.

Selective Serotonin Reuptake Inhibitors (SSRIs)

- This class of antidepressant medications has the same efficacy as the TCAs.

- SSRIs cause fewer side effects than the TCAs or MAO inhibitors.

- SSRIs do not cause hypotension, (Low blood pressure) sedation, or anticholinergic effects (e.g., confusion, blurred vision, constipation, dry mouth, light-headedness, difficulty starting and continuing to urinate, and loss of the bladder control), as do the TCAs.

- The reported side effects of the SSRIs are nausea, insomnia, sexual dysfunction and other mild side effect from each drug.

- All SSRIs have been found to be effective in the treatment of Obsessive-Compulsive Disorder (OCD).

Monoamine Oxidase Inhibitors (MAOIs)

- MAOIs are still used to treat Major Depression Disorder but only as a second or third choice.

- There is also the danger of taking MAOIs and other antidepressant medications.

- MAOIs decrease the amount on monoamine oxidase in the liver, which breakdown the amino acids of tyramine and tryptophan.

- MAOIs have some dangerous side effect such

as hypertensive crisis (e.g., elevated blood pressure, severe headache, severe anxiety, shortness of breath) when a person ingests tryamine rich foods (e.g., alcohol beverages, cheese, fruits, process foods, fish, soy, nuts and chocolates).

Chapter 6: Alternative Therapies and Complementary Therapies

Alternative and Complementary Therapies

Alternative therapies are often used for depression, fatigue, insomnia and anxiety. The most commonly used alternative therapies are as follows:

- Transcranial Magnetic Stimulation (TMS)

- Vagus Nerve Stimulation (VNS)

- St. John's Wort

- SAMe

- Tyrosine

- Vitamin B12

- Melatonin

- DHEA

- Omega-Fatty Acids

- Aromatherapy

- Acupuncture

Transcranial Magnetic Stimulation (TMS)

Transcranial Magnetic Stimulation (TMS) is the use of a magnetic field that passes through the skull, which cause cells in the cerebral cortex to fire. TMS has a rapid onset of action of (1 to 2 weeks), which is faster than most psychotropic medications. ECT and TMS have the same effectiveness in depression without psychosis, while depression with psychosis is best treated with ECT (Fontaine, 2003).

Vagus Nerve Stimulation (VNS)

Vagus Nerve Stimulation (VNS) has been used successfully with hard to treat seizure disorders and has FDA approval for this use. Recently, studies have focused on studying VNS for depression. A cookies side generator is placed in the chest under the skin that conveys electrical impulses via a connecting wire to the vagus nerve. (George, Nahas, Bohning, Mu, Kozel, Borckhart, & Denslow, 2004).

The nerve is the leading provider of the heart to the brain and other organs. VHS affects areas of the brain involved with mood. It provides continuous therapy (8 to 12 years), which is the life of the battery (Perraud, 2000).

St. John's Wort

St. John's (hypericum perforatum) has been the most widely publicized alternative treatment for mild and moderate depression. The side effects for St. John's Wort in higher dosages are similar to that of the SSRIs. It has been found to reduce the effectiveness of birth control pills, HIV treatment medications and the asthma medication-theophylline (Linde, Ramirer, Mulrow, Paula, Weidenhammer, et al., 1996).

SAMe

A nutritional supplement called SAMe (pronounced "sammy") has been used by more than 1 million people in Europe, primary for depression and arthritis. SAMe (S-adenosylmethionine), a compound made by every cell in the body, help produce DA, 5-HT and NE (Brown & Gerburg, 2000). It has been founded to be effective in depression, post-partum depression and postpartum menopausal depression. It may worsen with Bipolar Depression Disorder. Its rapid onset (10 to 12 days), low side effects (no weight gain or sexual dysfunction) and ability to boost antioxidants give it many advantages in the treatment of depression. Like the Tricylic antidepressants, SAMe should be used with causation in people who have a history of cardiac arrhythmia. Infants have (3 to 4 times) higher levels of SAMe than adults. Breast-feeding mother should be cognizant of the amount of SAMe passing through breast milk (Brown & Gerburg, 2000).

Tyrosine

Tyrosine is an amino acid and precursor for dopamine (DA) and norespinephrine (NE), which acts as a mood elevator. Supplemental tyrosine has been used in depression, stress reduction, anxiety and chronic fatigue. People taking MAO inhibitors should not take a supplements containing tyrosine because it may lead to hypertensive crisis. Tyrosine combined with vitamin B6 and Vitamin C will provide better absorption (Fontaine, 2003).

Vitamin B12

Vitamin B12 is necessary for norespinephrine (DA-5HT), and noespinephrine (NE) as well for the nature of synthesis of SAMe. Depression can cause lower levels through decreased appetite and resulting in decrease food intake. Many of the Tricyclic antidepressants deplete the body for Vitamin B12 (Fontaine, 2003).

Metatonin

Metatonin is a hormone secreted by the pineal gland. It plays a critical role in the regulation of the day-night cycle. Metatonin is effective in inducing sleep and has no notable side effects. Slow-release melatonin combined with standard antidepressant treatment often improves the sleep pattern in depressed individuals (Fontaine, 2003).

DHEA

Dehydroepiandrosterone (DHEA) is a corticosteriods produced primary in the adrenal glands. It serves as a precursor to testosterone and estrogen. DHEA may be involved in regulating mood and one sense of well-being. The method of action is unclear but it may stimulate GABA receptors or increase serotonin (5-HT levels). It has been used alone or in adjunct to antidepressants. Little is known about long risk of taking DHEA, however, it is best used under medical supervision. The usual dose is up to 90 mg daily (Wolkowitz, 1999).

Omega-3 Fatty Acids

Omega-3 Fatty Acids are derived from fish oils. They are thought to act on cells similar to Lithium, block calcium channels, as do the other mood stabilizers, and help regulate serotonin (5-HT). It appears to be an antidepressant, antimanic and a mood stabilizer. Research reported lower levels of Omego-3 level fatty acids in depression and the lower the levels, the more severe the depression (Fontaine, 2003).

Aromatherapy

Aromatherapy is the inhaling of essential oils through the use of a diffuser or using essential oils in massage. It may be beneficial in relieving depressive symptoms. The oils most often used are as follows: bergamot, geranium jasmine, lemon balm, rose, and ylang-ylang (Keville & Green, 1995; Snyder& Lindquist, 2006).

Acupuncture

Acupuncture is helpful in relieving feelings of depression and anxiety related to the rise in endorphin levels as a result of the treatment. Adding electrostimulation to acupuncture needles usually increases the effectiveness of treatment. After a single session, many people report a sense of well -being. It is unclear how helpful acupuncture is for Manic Depression/ Bipolar Disorder. Client response appears to be quite variable at the present time (Gerber, 2000).

Other Alternative and Complementary Therapies

Other alternative and complementary therapies are spiritual and therapeutic techniques used by clinicians with clients for healing for mental, spiritual and physical healing. Some of alternative and complementary interventions are as follows:

- Prayer

- Meditation

- Music Therapy

- Art Therapy

- Dance

- Literature

- Humor

- Relaxation

- Exercise

- Yoga

- Animal Assisted Therapy

- Therapeutic Massage

- Therapeutic Touch

Prayer

Prayer is communication with God or superior being. It can be individual or group action, or intercessory, which means conducted by other people without the knowledge of the individual (Snyder& Lindquist, 2006). The "laying on hands" and anointing the ill person with oil while praying for healing is an ancient form of intercessory prayer (Fortinash & Holoday-Worret, 2000). Using spirituality principles such as biblical scriptures (e.g., meditation on scriptures), belief in a higher power, spiritual teachings for healing are used for spiritual healing. Certain religious groups used prayer and meditation as a mean of spiritual healing.

Meditation

Meditation techniques include a routine time and place, assuming a comfortable position, using deep breathing and progression relaxation exercise and focusing on mental image. The relaxation response to meditation consists of a wide range of beneficial

physiologic and psychological effects, including heart
and blood pressure rates, decreased serum levels of
adrenal corticosteriods, increased immunity to disease,
a sense of calmness and peace and mental health alertness (Fortinash & Holoday-Worret, 2000).

Music Therapy

Music therapy includes the use of specific kinds of
music and its ability to effect changes in behavior, emotions, and physiology. Music is often used in intensive
care units, birthing room, during dental procedures,
and even stimulus for people with lower levels of consciousness. Music therapy impacted on positive health
outcomes in research studies (e.g., decreased pain;
decreased stress) (Fortinash & Holoday-Worret, 2000;
Snyder& Lindquist, 2006).

Art Therapy

Art has been used with children and adults for the
expression of their feelings about stressful situations
and consciousness concern about their illnesses.   It
can produce a calming effect. Art expression has been
a psychotherapy tool in geriatric centers, children and
adolescents, in hospice, alcohol treatment programs
and in prisons (Rubin, 1998).

Dance

Dance is an expression of joy and celebration
throughout the world. It has been used as a means
to increase self-esteem and body image, lesser depression, fear, isolation and express emotions even anger
(Fortinash & Holoday-Worret, 2000).

Literature

Books, poetry, and religious writings can be inspirational and can cause a person to become immersed for long periods in reading. Journal and diaries are also forms of expressing one's emotions and have been referred to as a "process of meditation" and conversation with the self (Fortinash & Holoday-Worret, 2000).

Humor

Humor and laughter are also used for expressing emotions, for relieving tension and anxiety, and coping with pain and unpleasant situations. Laughter has positive effects on respiratory, heart rates, blood pressure and muscle tension (Fortinash & Holoday-Worret, 2000;
Snyder& Lindquist, 2006).

Relaxation

Relaxation therapy has had a positive impact on health outcomes and it is psychophysiological state characterized by parasympathetic dominance involving multiple visceral and somatic symptoms, including the absence of physical, mental and emotional tension (Snyder& Lindquist, 2006). Progressive relaxation needs to be practiced twice a day for 20 minutes. It will be weeks before a person experiences the benefits of this technique (Fortinash & Holoday-Worret, 2000; Snyder& Lindquist, 2006).

Exercise

The benefits of physical exercise are well known. It can bring a general sense of well -being and vitality, increase respiratory and cardiovascular efficiency and promote longer life. Exercise raises levels of endorphins, which enhance one's feelings of well -being.   Exercise also increases levels of dopamine (DA), Serotonin -5-HT, and norespinephrine (NE), which are feelings of rewards, motivation and attention (Snyder& Lindquist, 2006; Steptoe, 2006).

Yoga

Living a balanced life is central to yoga principles. The use of specific body postures, breathe control, minimizing stimulation of the senses, leading a simple life, and directed meditation are achieved through daily practices (Feuerstein, 2001; Snyder& Lindquist, 2006).

Animal Assisted Therapy

Companionship with animals is associated with people experiencing less depression and loneliness. Animals provide meaningful and substantial comfort for many individuals. The research has reported elderly women who are more at risk for depression, who live alone to be in better emotional health if they lived with an animal. They were less lonely, more optimistic, and more interested in the future than women who lived alone without a pet (Hart, 2000; Snyder& Lindquist, 2006).

Therapeutic Massage

More than 80 difference forms of massage therapies have been identified. These forms vary from gentle stroking to deep kneading, rubbing and percussion. Most massage is done with the hands. The primary purpose of massage therapy is to result in muscle and total body relaxation and increased circulation.   Extensions of massage technique involve deep tissue and advanced massage techniques; of the skin and underlying tissues for the purposes of increasing circulation and inducing a relaxation response   (Fortinash & Holoday-Worret, 2000; Snyder& Lindquist, 2006).

Therapeutic Touch (TT)

Healing through touch can be traced back to early civilization.   Nurses have practiced various forms of therapeutic touch for many years.   The benefits of contact touch such as message have been recently identified as providing a sense of spiritual balance, relieving mental and emotional tension and anxiety, improving blood flow, easing pain, and stimulating the immune system.   Also, therapeutic touch refers to a noncontact technique derived from the "laying on hands" associated with Eastern, European, and religious philosophies. This method is based on a theory that the release of energy from the healer assists the ill person in the healing process (Fortinash & Worret, 2000; Snyder& Lindquist, 2006).

Chapter 7: Depression and Medical Treatment

Misdiagnosis

Often, depression in women is misdiagnosed and approximately (30-50 %) prescriptions for antidepressants are given to women (Greenberg et al., 1993). Women have the highest utilization of medical services (Becker & Newson, 2003). There is an over utilization of emergency department with (a) emotional problems, (b) suicidal attempts and (c) high use of days lost from work related to depression (Becker & Newsom, 2003; Bender, 2005; Greenberg et al., 1993). Increase incidence of depression is seen in primary care and hospital settings. Major depression is one of the most common clinical problems encountered by primary care practitioners (Zung, Broadhead, & Roth, & 1993). It accounts for more bed days (people of work and in bed) than other physical disorder except cardiovascular disorders. It is more costly to the economy than chronic respiratory illness, diabetes, arthritis, or hypertension (Greenberg et al., 1993). Depression is often denied or not identity by patients. Healthcare professional may not assess or identify depressive symptoms (Greenberg et al., 1993). It is estimated that depression cost the American economy $43.7 billion worker absenteeism, lost productivity and health care (Greenberg et al., 1993).

Depression often has been misdiagnosed in African American community (Carrington, 2006; Coridan & O'Connell, 2002). Factors that can contribute fewer African Americans being diagnosed with clinical depression include.

- A mistrust of medical health professionals, based on part of historical higher than average institutionalization for African American with mental illness

- Cultural barriers, influenced by language and values in relationship between doctors and the patient

- Reliance on the support of family and the religious community, rather than mental health professional, during periods of emotional distress

- A masking of depressive symptoms by other medical conditions, somatic complaints, substance abuse and other psychiatric illnesses

- Socioeconomic factors, such as limited access to medical care (NMHA, 2004)

Some women may deny or not identify their depressed moods but report a variety of somatic complaints (Stuart & Laraia, 2001). These somatic complaints may include gastrointestinal distress, chronic or intermittent pain, irritability, palpitation, dizziness, appetite change, lack of energy, change in sex drive, or sleep disturbance. Women often focus on somatic symptoms because they are more sociably acceptable than the feeling of sadness, inability to concentrate, or loss of pleasure in usual activities (Stuart & Laraia, 2001).

Although (10 to 15 %) of pregnant women meet the criteria for depression, they often remain undiagnosed because of the symptoms of depression are similar to the somatic changes of pregnancy. The prevalence of depression among pregnant adolescent is almost twice as high as among adult pregnant women and is more severe between the second and third trimesters. Untreated maternal depression is associated with poor prenatal delivery, small infant size, postpartum depression, and maternal suicide (Szigethy & Ruiz, 2001).

Depression and Medical Conditions

The research has revealed a high incidence of depression among hospitalized patients from medical conditions (Gottlieb, Khatta, Friedmann, Einbinder, Katzen, Baker, et. al., 2004). Depression rates among hospitalized patients range from (13% to 77.5%); outpatient research studies have been less   rates of (13% to 42%) (NIMH, 2008).

Often these depressive symptoms are unrecognized and thus are untreated by healthcare professionals (NIMH, 2008).   African American women often access inpatient and the Emergency Room for health care for treatment (Becker & Newsom, 2003).   These health services organizations are primary areas for assessment of depression and for making appropriate referrals.

Depression is found in all severities of medical conditions (Becker & Newsom, 2003; NMHA, 2004).   The intensity and frequencies of depression are highest in more severely ill patients (NMHA, 2004). Approximately, one third of hospitalized patients reports symptoms of mild or moderate symptoms of depression and one fourth may have a depressive illness (NMHA, 2004). Medical conditions associated with depression are cancer, cardiac disease, and a variety of endocrine disorders (Bender, 2005; Martin, 2003; NIMH, 2008). African American women have numerous physical health problems, (Stuart & Laraia, 2001). However, more research studies are needed on the relationship of African American women and health outcomes (Scarinic, Beech, & Watson, 2004).

In addition, the research has reported depression as common in patients with heart failure, with age, gender, and race influencing its prevalence in ways similar to those observed in the general population (Gottlieb,

Khatta, Friedmann, Einbinder, Katzen, Baker, et. al., 2004).

Obesity is prevalence among African American women (Bender, 2005). It has been positively associated with depression in African American women (Garvin, Williams, Siefert, & Hastings, 2003).

However, few studies have focused specifically on the relationship between obesity and depressive symptoms in African American women

(Gavin, Williams, Siefert, & Hastings, 2003). There has been an increase of Type 2 Diabetes in African American women. Women with Type 2 Diabetes experience long periods of depression due, impart to a lack of economic and social resources (Martin, 2003). Also, environmental exposure or hazardous chemical is often associated with poor health outcomes. Researchers have neglected to understand the impact of the environment on African American women's mental health (Hastings, Williams & Jackson, 2003). A study by Hastings, Williams & Jackson (2003) reported that African American women exposed to environmental hazards reported higher symptoms of distress when experiencing discrimination (29 %) and were (4 times) as likely to be experience a distress when married. Both white and African American women showed that not having health insurance increase depression and psychological distress without exposure to hazardous environments. Also, poor African Americans are disproportionately represented among households experiencing insufficiency. An inadequate household food supply associated with depression among low-income women (Siefert, Heflin, & William, 2003). One study reported that African American women with depression symptoms were much more likely to engage in HIV-associated risk behavior than African American women without the depressive symptoms. These women reported greater risk exposure through sexual partners (Focus, 1995).

Historically, mental health professionals have consistently underdiagnosed depression and overdiagnosed schizophrenia in the African American community (Coridan & O'Connell, 2002; DeCoux Hampton, 2007). In addition to socioeconomic factors, African American women have limited access to health care compared to white women (Coridan & O' Connell, 2002; Mitchell & Herring 2003). Many African American women have problem with access to proper care and insurance limiting them from receiving treatment for depression (Bender, 2005; The Common Wealth Fund, 2002). However, when they seek mental health care it is usually later in life or when the condition is in the late stage.

Outpatient Management

Depression is prevalence in primary care settings (Becker & Newsom, 2003). Approximately, (1 out of 5) patients seeing a primary care practitioner have significant symptoms of depression. However only about (1 in 100 patients) reported depression as the reason for the most recent visit. Healthcare providers fail to diagnose Major Depression Disorder in their patients up to (50 %) of the time (Zung, Broad, & Broth, 1993). Primary care physicians are less likely to detect signs of depression in African American women. However, primary care is in a key position to assess depression of African American women. They could have significant impact on minority patients overall access to mental health care because of adequate assessment for depression and appropriate referrals.

African American women may access inpatient and outpatients with health problem, which may be related to undiagnosed depression. Also, these primary care health services organizations are more cultural acceptable places to seek health care for African Americans than mental health organizations.

Access to Care

Despite the life expectancy for African Americans rising substantially in the last fifty years, the rate of mortality, disease and disability among blacks continues to be greater than whites (Becker & Newsom, 2003). The death rate for African Americans is (1.6 times) higher than whites. In addition, statistics reports include (8 out of the 10 leading causes of death) are associated with a higher mortality rate for blacks as compared to whites (Becker & Newsom, 2003). African Americans are also less likely to be covered by health insurance and have health insurance. Research indicates that the access to health care is also bureaucratized which leads to patient satisfaction that is differential. Of all ethnic groups, African Americans are the most likely to depend on health care services that are hospital based such as emergency rooms and ambulatory clinics (Becker & Newsom, 2003; Bender, 2005). The overuse of hospitals results in decrease quality of care since patients do not have their own physicians to build a trusting relationship and to monitor their health, which in turn reinforces their mistrust in the health care system. Dissatisfaction in the health care system along with mistrust results in a deterrent for seeking health care (Becker & Newsom, 2003). So, depression may not be diagnosed or treated in this group.

Chapter 8: Strategies for Improvement

The proposed strategies in improving treatment for African Americans women are (a) developing and using more practical, reliable and valid scales for measuring depression, (b) assessing adequately for depression in African American women (e.g., using cultural sensitive tools for gathering data and obtaining histories and physicals (H&Ps), (c) providing culture sensitive treatment, (d) involving community (e.g., church, community centers, etc.) in treatment issues for depressed African American women, (e) educating healthcare providers on cultural competent treatment and care and (h) mentoring of African American women by other African American women. These issues will be addressed individually. Please refer to Table 1, page 72.

Table 1: Conceptual Model of Strategies for Improving Depression in African Americans Women

Biopsychosocial-Spiritual Factors

Variables	Concepts	Strategies for Improvement
Sociodemograhic Factors • Environmental Factors • Socioeconomic Factors • Health Factors • Cultural Factors	**Psychosocial Factors** • Stress Factors + - • Coping Skills Factors + - • Social Support Factors + -	**Interventions** • Developing Cultural Sensitive Tool/Practical Reliable and Valid Scales for Depression • Assessing Adequately for Depression (e.g., using Cultural Assessment Tools. • Providing Cultural Sensitive Treatment • Involving Community in Treatment Issues • Educating Healthcare professionals on Culture Competent Treatment and Care • Mentoring of African American Women by other African American Women

Health Outcomes

Cultural Sensitive Tools

Researchers need to develop more reliable, practical, and valid tools to measure depression in African American and other minority groups (Zasuzniewski et al., 2002). Tools for assessing depression need to be cultural sensitive. Focus groups are excellent means of gathering data to develop tools. Also, healthcare professionals providing care for African American women need to share their experiences with others in the most effective treatment regimens in treating this population. Also, healthcare professionals need to be aware of cultural factors when conducting assessment and obtaining a medical history and physical (H&P).

Adequate Assessment for Depression

Healthcare providers working with African Americans need to frequently assess African American women for depression. A cultural assessment would be a useful tool in data gathering. Often, it is difficult to treat mental health problems in African American women. Health care providers often are less likely to detect diagnosable mental disorders in African Americans (Miranda & Cooper 2004). The complexity of their treatment issues has had a negative impact on health outcomes. One reason is that African American women tend to minimize the serious nature of their problems. A second reason is that many believe their problem is just the blues and they are not proactive in changing their condition. A third reason is there is a stigma placed on mental health problems in the African American culture that they are a sign of weakness, not a sickness. They often feel they can take care of the problem on their own (Mitchell & Herring, 2003). In addition, African Americans often delay or will not seek treatment for depression (Black, 2001).

Clinical depression is often a vague disorder for

African American women (Warren, 1995). White women reports more "typical symptoms" of depression such as e.g., depressed mood while African American women reports more somatic symptoms of depression. When African American women do access the healthcare system, they are assessed for the physical symptoms and may not be assess for depression. The origins of their symptoms are not explored. These women continue to complain of being tired, weary, empty, lonely and sad. However, African American women are less likely to take antidepressant medications when prescribed (Miranda & Cooper, 2004).

Often, African American women may be misdiagnosed because they go to health care visits looking well-groomed regardless of feeling depressed or sad. As a result, healthcare professionals often see their appearance as well- groomed, not disheveled during their assessment. When assessing African American females, they often deny feeling depressed because they don't want to be seen as weak or not spiritually strong. In some culture, common phrases of African American women when referring to their health problems are "I am not going to claim it" or "I 'm bless." Historically, mental health professionals have consistently underdiagnosed disorder e.g., depression and overdiagnosed disorders like schizophrenia in the African American community.

Cultural Sensitive Treatment

Often, when African American women seek counseling, she is admitting she is not handling her problem well. In addition, she is admitting she has a problem and validating lack of self-control. African American women may feel they are giving up power and may not want to be vulnerable when acknowledging feeling depressed (Black, 2003).

Current treatments for depression include

psychotherapy, somatic or physical therapies and medications (Das & Weissman, 2006). Psychotherapies and medications have reported to improve depression in minority women (Miranda, Chung, Green, Krupnick, Siddique, et al., 2003).

African American women need to understand that depression is not a weakness, but an illness often resulting from a combination of causes. Antidepressants are useful for treating   chemical imbalances or physical disorders. Psychotherapy is effective for depression. However, certain surgeries or certain heart, hormonal, blood pressure, or kidney medications may actually induce the symptoms of depression. African American women may require being more sensitivity to certain antidepressants and smaller dosages than traditional treatment advises (McGrath et al., 1992).

Psychotherapies should address issues of   competing roles, lack of opportunities, lack of skilled,   managerial jobs and low paying wages,   etc. The focus of psychotherapies needs to address such issues as correcting conflict,   correcting interpersonal conflict and developing interpersonal skills. Couple therapy needs to be used to reduce relationship conflict.

In addition, psychotherapy or group therapy needs to focus on identifying the cause of depression, the treatment of choice, enhancing self-esteem, and developing alternative strategies in order to handle their stress and conflicting roles appropriately. African American women need to learn relaxation techniques, and develop alternative coping and crisis strategies. Group sessions are excellent forums for African American women because of the support and the wider selections of lifestyle choice and changes. Self-help groups may provide social support for depressed African American women to enhance the work accomplished in therapeutic settings (Warren, 1995).

Cognitive therapy focuses on removing symptoms by

identifying and correcting negative behavior. For example, African Americans women's perception of racism or discrimination may cause " oppression or negative behaviors " resulting in depressive symptoms. In order to correct these negative behaviors they must change their negative perceptions of life situations by developing a **sense of empowerment.** In addition, the stigma associated with seeking mental and emotional health prevents many African women from admitting they are struggling with these issues and identifying alternative solutions. Therapists need to assist African American women in identifying and exploring more positive alternative strategies in   problem- solving.

For many African American women spirituality is necessary in the concept of healing for depression. Spirituality creates attitudes that embrace hope and empowerment. In a healthy person, spirituality is critical for overall mental health using the network found in the family, neighborhood, church, mosque, temple and community (Mitchell & Herring, 2003).

The education of African American women on depression is crucial. African Americans women must put forth an effort to be successful by overcoming fears. They must recognize symptoms of depression. No two people experience mental problems in the same way. Symptoms may vary in severity and duration among difference people. For example, a feeling of worthless is a common sign of depression in white women and change of appetite is a common symptom of depression in black women.

Organizations in the African American community e.g. church groups, schools, health departments, community centers, sororities, etc., need to provide more support and resources for African American women. For example, support groups are excellent forums for African American women to deal with psychosocial issues. African American women seek healing through other women with similar experiences.

African American women seek mental health services far less frequent as white women (Das & Weissman, 2006; Miranda & Cooper, 2004). They often engage in informal sources of help, such as prayer or having "sister support group" and talk with friends in hope of gaining what other may gain in individual therapy (Black, 2001). Independent support for black women is being created around the country. Also, in supportive settings such as support groups, church affiliation groups (e.g., women ministries), available resources etc. need to be provided to assist with mental health services, financial support etc. African American women tend to rely on these groups rather than mental health services etc. They tend to use networks such as friends, family, churches etc., to help them cope (Steven, 1998). The involvement of organizations in their communities may be helpful in identifying depression, access to the appropriate health services and treatment of African American women for depression. These strategies are particularly helpful because when they seek mental health care it is usually later in life or when the condition is in the late stage.

Spirituality needs to be considered in treatment of African American women. Abrums (2004) explores how women from an African American congregation respond to oppression in healthcare. Data from interviews describe experiences related to health, personal religious devotion, and racism. The experiences are categorized by four different themes: 1) the meaning of intelligence versus education, 2) the power of prayer, 3) the demonstration of agency in healthcare encounters and 4) the role of Jesus in healthcare (p. 194). Overall, the women express resistance to oppression and racism encountered in the healthcare system through personal relationships with God and Jesus and through support and strength found within the church congregation. The women in this study emphasized the influence of a personal belief in **Jesus,** focusing on **His presence and His power,** on health and **resistance to negative experiences within the healthcare system.**

Another main theme discussed by Abrums (2004) focused on supportive relationships in the church. Church leaders and members affirmed the worth and value of one another, thereby supporting one another in healthcare encounters. Overriding all themes was the idea of **Jesus as the true Healer.** In this context, the healthcare system was seen as a tool the **Lord** could use in the process of healing as opposed to an ultimate authority.

Cultural Sensitive Education for HealthCare Providers

Healthcare professionals who especially provide care to African American population need to take the lead in educating the public on healthcare issues of African American population e.g., health disparities, treatment, consultation, etc. There is a need for more conferences, workshops etc. related to assessing cultural competent care of African Americans and other minority groups.

Healthcare professionals need to be educated on identifying common symptoms of depression in African American women. Their cultural barriers may be influenced by language and values in relationship between healthcare providers and the clients. Some women may deny or not identify their depressed moods but report a variety of somatic complaints e.g. gastrointestinal distress, chronic or intermittent pain, irritability, palpitation, dizziness, appetite change, lack of energy, change in sex drive, or sleep disturbance. They often focus on these symptoms because they are more sociably acceptable than the feeling of sadness, inability to concentrate, or loss of pleasure in usual activities (Stuart & Laraia, 2004).

Health care professionals need to know the language of African American. Less than (10 %) of African Americans suffering from depression seek help (Black, 2003). Cultural barriers, including in the presentation of symptoms may influence language and behavior mannerisms (Barbee, 1992).

In a study of African American women with depression, Barbee reported that the language of depression differed from health professionals' nomenclature and the distinctive language of depression. African American women were constructed around the cultural symbol of blues music. African American world-views are concerned with family and group survival in American society. This worldview emphasizes one's spirituality, interdependence within element of the universe with less emphasis placed on material goods. This worldview may have some bearing on African American women's ways of experiencing depression (Amankwaa, 2003).

Communicating to African American women by healthcare professionals need to be culturally sensitive. Scarinic, Beech, and Watson (2004) examined the relationship between physicians- interaction and depression among African American women. Depression was positively associated with difficulty talking with physicians, likelihood of discussing problems with physicians, reporting physician had made offensive comments. In addition, they were more likely to change physicians due to dissatisfaction.

Mentoring

Mentoring of African American women with other African American women is essential in for preventing life issues causing depression. For example, African American women in leadership positions need to mentor and support other African American women in career development. Mentors are very critical for African American women in terms of career development and support system. In a qualitative study of (14) African-American women on an interview indicated that mentoring was very important to their career development. Barriers in obtaining traditional mentoring in their organizations were (a) stereotypes of African American women and (b) racism (Bova, 1998). The mentoring in the workplace focused more on the career development aspects of their life and that they received psychosocial support which was critical for their career success, from groups they affiliated with throughout their lives. For the African American women, mentoring may take place in other settings other than the workplace. Organization such as church groups, schools, sororities, community centers are excellent places for forming mentoring groups for African American women.

Health Outcomes

The author proposed that the *Conceptual Model of Strategies for Improving Depression in African Americans Women* is a framework to conceptualize cultural sensitive strategies for improving health outcomes. The model will be a useful framework for providing treatment and conducting research related to depression and African American women.

Conclusion

More research studies are needed to examine the relationship of certain sociodemographic factors and psychosocial factors e.g., stress, coping, social support of depression in African American women and health outcomes. Depression is found in all severities of medical conditions. African American women have numerous medical problems and psychosocial factors, in addition to a higher incidence of depression than other races. Often, depressions in African American women are undiagnosed or misdiagnosed and there is a cultural stigma in the African American community for mental health treatment, which prevents access and compliance to treatment.   Health care professionals need to provide more culture sensitive treatment related to diagnosis, and interventions for African American women with depression. Researchers need to development more culture sensitive assessment tools. In addition, health care professionals need to educate the public on the culture perspective in the identification of depression in African American women. Also, social support groups and mentoring are excellent strategies in building a support system for African American women.

References

Abrums, M. (2004). Faith and feminism: How African American women from a storefront church resist oppression in health care. *Advances in Nursing Science, 27*(3), 187-201.

Alexander, J.L. (2007). Quest for timely detection treatment of women with depression. *Journal of Managed Care Pharmacy*, 3-11.

Amankwaa, L. .C. (2003, Spring) . Postpartum depression, culture and

African American Women. *Journal of Cultural Diversity* 1-2.

American Psychiatric Association (2000). Diagnostic and Statistical Manual of Mental Disorders   (4th ed.). Washington, DC.

Barbee, E. L. (1992). African-American women and depression: A review and critique of the literature. *Archives of Psychiatric Nursing*, 6(5), 257-265.

Barrow, G.   (2003). Fighting black female depression. *Sacramento Observer New   Report, Retrieved from Internet July 16, 2006, http://newsncmonline.com/ news/ view_article.htm? article_id.*

Becker, G., Newsom, E. (2003). Socioeconomic status and dissatisfaction with health care among chronically ill African Americans. *American Journal of Public Health, 96*, 742-748.

Belle, D. & Doucet, J. (2003). Poverty, inequality and discrimination as sources of depression among U.S. women. *Psychology of Women Quarterly,* 27 (2) 101-113.

Bender, E. (2005). Depression treatment in black women must consider social factors. *American Psychiatry News,* 40 (23), 14.

Bhatia , S.C. & Bhatia, S. K. (1999). Depression in women: Diagnostic and treatment consideration. *American Academy of Family,* 1-16.

Black, C. (2003). Silent Treatment- Many Black Women Struggle with Depression on Their Own. *Race and Ethnicity in the New Urban American* (Retrieved from Internet, 5/8/2003) http://www.jrn.columbia.edu/ studentwork/race/2001/ silent_black.shtml.

Bloch, M. Schmidt, P. J. Danaceau, M. Murphy, J. Nieman, L. & Rubinow, D.R. (2000). Effects of gonadal steroids in women with a history of postpartum depression. *American Journal of Psychiatry,* 157 (6) 924-930.

Blumenthal, R. & Endicott, J. (1996). Barriers to seeking treatment for Major   Depression. *Depression and Anxiety,* 4 (6), 281-284.

Bova, B. M. (1999). Mentoring Revisited The African American Women's   Experience. 1998 *AERC Proceedings.* Retrieved from Internet April 20 2006, http://www. edst.educ.ubc.ca/aerc/1998/98bova.htm.

Breslau, N. Kilbey, M. & Adreski, P. (1993). Nicotine dependence,   major depression, and anxiety in adults. *Archives General Psychiatry,* 50 31-35.

Brown, R.P. & Gerburg, P. L. (2000). Integrative psychop-harmacology. In P.P. Muskin (ED) *Complementary and Interactive Medicine and Psychiatry* (p.p. 1-66). Washington, D.C. American Psychiatric Press.11

Brown, S. & McNair, L. (1995). Black women's sexual sense of self: Implications for aids prevention. *Journal of Women Treatment and* Research, 1-8.

Carrington, C.H. (2006). Clinical depression in African American women: Diagnosis, treatment, and research. *Journal of Clinical Psychology*, 62 (7) 779 –791.

Cohen, L.S., Soares, C.H. & Joffe, H. (2005). Diagnosis and management of mood disorders during the meno-pausal transition. *American Journal of Medicine*, 118 (Suppl 2), 93-97.

Cohen, S. & Williamson, G. M. (1991). Stress and infec-tious disease. *Psychological Bulletin,* 109, 5-24.

Cohen, S. & Wills, T .A. (1985). Stress, social support, and the buffering hypothesis. *Psychological Bulleton,* 98 (2), 310-357.

Coridan, C. & O'Connell, C. (2002). Meeting the ending Treatment of Disparities for Women of Color-a back-ground paper. *National Mental Health Association,* http//www.ncstac.org/Meeting_the_Challenge. pdfPsychology Quarterly, 13 (3), 293-311.

Centers for Disease Control and Prevention (2007). National Center for Injury Prevention and Control. Web based Injury Statistics Query and Reporting System (WISQARS). Retrieved Jan. 3, 2007, from: http://www.cdc.gov/ncipc/wisqars.

Clark, R., Anderson, N. , B. Clark, V. R. & Williams, D. R. (1999). Racism as a stressor for African Americans, A Biopsycholocial Model. *American Psychologist*, 54 805-116.

Das, O. C. & Weissman, M. (2006). Depression in African American: Breaking barriers to detection and treatment: Community –based studies tend to ignore high-risk groups of African Americans. *Journal of Family Practice*, 15-21.

DeCoux Hampton, M. (2007). The role of treatment and high acuity in the overdiagnosis of Schizophrenic in African Americans. *Archives of Psychiatric Nursing*, 21 (6), 327-335.

Diagnostic and Statistical Manual of Mental Disorders (4th ed). (DSM-IV). (2000). Revised Book, American Psychiatric Press, Washington, D.C.

Early, K.E., & Akers, R.L. (1993). It's a white thing": An explanation of beliefs about suicide in the African American community. *Deviant Behavior, 14*, 227-96.

Feuerstein, G. (2001). *Yoga*, Holm Press.

Focus (1995, August). Risk and Depression in Black Women, 9,7.

Folkman, S. & Lazarus, R.S. (1980). An analysis of coping in the middle-aged community sample. *Journal of health and social behavior*, 21 (3), 219-239.

Fontaine, K. (2003). *Mental health nursing*. Prentice Hall Company.

Fortinash, K.M. & Holoday-Worret, P.A. (2003). *Psychiatric mental health* Mosby Company.

Frisch, N.C. & Frisch, L.E. (2006). *Psychiatric-mental health nursing* (3rd ed.). Delmar Publisher Company.

Garvin, A. R. Williams, D.R. Siefert, K., & Hastings, J.F. D. (2003). Obesity and Depression in African American Women. *African American Women and Depression: New Findings on a Neglected Topic*, NIMH Center for Research on Poverty, Risk, and Mental Health, Publisher Company 20-21.

Geber, R. (2000). *Vibrational medicine for the 21st century*, New York: Eagle Book.

George, M.S., Nahas, Z, Bohning, D.E., Mu, Q.,F., Kozel, A., Borckhart, J. & Denslow, S. (2004). Mechanism of action Vagus Nerve Stimulation. *Clinical Neuroscience Research*, 4 (1), 71-19.

Glied, S. & Kofman S. (1995, March). Women and Mental Health: Issues for Health Reform Background paper. New York, *The Commonwealth Fund Commission on Women Health.*

Goldsmith, S. K. (2001). *Risk factors for suicide: Summary of a workshop.* Washington, DC: National Academy Press

Gottlieb, S.S., Khatta, M., Friedmann, E., Einbinder, L., Katzen, S., Baker, B. et. al., (2004). The influence of age, gender, and race on the prevalence of depression in heart failure patients. *JACC,* 43:1542-1549.

Greenburg, P. et al., (1993). The economic burdened depression in 1990, *Journal of Clinical Psychiatry,* 54, 28.

Griffith, L.S. & Lustaman, P.J. (1997). Depression in women with Diabetes. *Diabetes Spectrum,* 10 (2), 216-223.

Hart, L.A. (2000). Psychosocial benefits of animal companionship. In A.H. Fine (ED). *Handbook on animal-assisted therapy* (p.p. 59-78), San Diego: Academic Press.

Hastings, J.F., Williams, D.R. & Jackson, W. J. (2003). Exposure to Environmental Hazards: A Link to Depression and Psychological Distress Among African American Women, *African American Women and Depression: New Findings on A Neglected Topic,* NIMH Center for Research, Poverty, Risk, and Mental Health.

Jesse, E. , Walcott-Quigg, M., A. & Swanson, M. (2005). Risk and protective factors associated with symptoms of depression in low income African American with Causasian women during pregnancy.

Journal of Midwifery & Women's Health, 50 (5), 405-410.

Joe, S., et al (2006). Prevalence of and risk factors for lifetime suicide attempts among blacks in the United States. *Journal of American Medical Association,* 296 (17), 2112-2113.

Jones, L. V. (2002). *Intervening with Black women at-risk of depression: An Innovative psycho-educational group approach.* Ijones@albany.edu.

Jones, I. & Craddock, N. (2001). Familiarity of the puerperal trigger in bipolar disorder. *American Journal of Psychiatry,* 158 (6) 913-917.

Jones-Webb, R. & Snowden, L. (1993). Symptoms of depression among blacks and whites. *American Journal of Public Health,* 83, 240.

Keith, V. M. and Norwood, R. S. (1997). Marital strain and Depressive Symptoms among African American. *African American Research Perspectives,* 3 (2), 7-11.

Kennedy, B. K. (2009). Psychosocial Model: Racism as predictor of adherence and compliance to treatment and health outcomes with African Americans. *Journal of Theory Construction & Testing,* 13 (1), 20-26.

Kennedy, B.R., Mathis, C.C. & Woods, A. (2007). African American and their distrust of the health care system: Healthcare for diverse populations. *Journal of Cultural Diversity: An Interdisciplinary Journal,* 14 (2), 56-60.

Keville, K. & Green, M. (1995). *Aromatherapy: A complete guide to the art of healing. The Crossing Press.*

Kopelman, C., Moel, J., Mertens, C. Stuart, S. Arndt, S. & O'Hara, W. (2008). Barriers to care for antenatal depression. *Psychiatric Services,* 59 (4), 429.

LaVeist, T. A. (2000). Race Ethnicity, and Health. A Public Health Reader, Jossey- Bass Company.

Linde, K. Ramirer, G. Mulrow, C.D. Pauls, A. Weidenhammer, W. & Melchart, D. (1996). St John's Wort for depression. An overview and meta-analysis of randomized clinical trials. *British Medical Journal,* 313, 1065-1066.

Leven, A. (2003, July). Psychotherapy; Medication most effective to fight minority women depression. *Health Behavior New Service* or www.hbns.org.

Martin, J. (2003). High rates of depression found in African American women at risk for type 2 diabetes. *Washington University in St Louis New Information,* School of Medicine, (Retrieved from Internet 5-8-2006), http://mednews.wustl.edu/tips/page/normal/592.html.

McGrath, E., Keita, G.P., Strickland, B. R. & Russo, N. F. (1990). Women and depression: Risk factors and treatment issues. *American Psychological Association,* Hyattsville, MD.

Mills, T. L. (2000). *Depression, Mental and psychosocial well-being among older African Americans: A selective review of the literature.* Department of Sociology, University of Florida.

Miranda, J. Chung, J.Y., Green, B.L. , Krupnick, J., Siddique, J. et al., (2003). Treating depression in predominantly low-income young minority women. *JAMA,* 290, 57-65.

Miranda, J. & Cooper, L., A. (2004). Disparities in care for depression among primary care patients. *Journal of General Internal Medicine,* 471-485.

Mitchell, A. & Herring, K. (2003). *Black women overcoming stress and Depression.* BlackwomensHealth.Com.

National Institute of Mental Health (NIMH) (2008). Retrieved from The Internet from http://www.nimh.nih.gov/about/index.shtmlom.

.*National Mental Health Association* (2004). Clinical Depression and African Americans. Alexandria, VA.

Pajer, K. (1995). New strategies in the treatment of depression in Women. *Journal of Clinical Psychiatry,* 56 (Suppl. 2), 30-37.

Perraud, S. (2000). Efforts intensify to treat chronic depression. *Nurse Week,* Retrieved from Internet 10/17/2008 from http://www2.nursingspectum.com/articles/article.cfm?aid=3602

Research Agenda for Psychosocial and Behavioral Factors in Women's Health (1996, February), Washington Women Program Office, American Psychological Association.

Roco, C. (2005). Women's Programs, National Institute of Mental Health National Institutes of Health (NIH). Retrieved from 10/18/2008 from http://www.4women.gov/FAQ/postpartum.htm#7

Rouse, D., L. (2001). Lives of women of color create risk for depression. *Women's News* (Retrieved from Internet, 5/8/2006), http://www.womensenews.org/article.cfm/dyn/aid/666.

Rubin, J.A. (1998). *Art therapy/Moral and ethical aspect.* Psychology Press.

Santoro, N.F., & Green, R. (2009). Menopause symptoms and ethnicity: lessons from the study of women's health across the national. *Menopause Medicine,* 17 (1) , Retrieved from Internet, Feburary 28, 2009., from http://www.srm-ejournal.com/article.asp?AID=7294

Scarinic, I. C. Beech, B. M. A., & Watson, J. M. (2004). Physician -patient interaction and depression among African – American women: A national study. *Ethnicity & Disease,* 14 (4) 567-573.

Siefert, K. Heflin, C. M. & Williams, D. R. (2003). Household Food Insufficiency and Depression in African American and Women. *African American Women and Depression: A New Finding on A neglected Topic*, NIMH Center for Research on Poverty, Risk, and Mental Health.

Sigelman, L. & Welch, S. (1991). *Black Americans views of racial inequality: The Dream Deferred. Cambridge*, M.A, and Harvard University Press.

Snyder, R.L & Lindguist, R. (2006). *Complimentary/alternative therapies in nursing.* Springfield Publication Company.

Steptoe, A. (2006). *Depression, mental /physiological aspect,* Cambridge University Press.

Steven. C. (1998). *Support Network May Help Black Women Cope Better With   Depression. University of Florida Show*, Retrieved from Internet 5-28-2006, http://www.sciencedaily.com/releases/1998/07/980715140746.htm.

Stewart, P. E. (2004). Afrocentric approaches to working with African American Families in Society. *The Journal of Contemporary Social Services*, (85) 2, 221-228.

Stock, M. (2005). *Depression: What Every Woman Should Know. 2005 National* Institute of Health (NIMH) NIH Publication No. 05-4779. www.nimh.nih.gov/publicat/depwomenknows.cfm.

Stuart, G. W. & Laraia, M. T. (2001). *Principles of psychiatric nursing* (6th ed.). Mosby Company.

Sue, D. W., & Sue, D. (2005). *Ethnic and cultural awareness* (4th ed.). Hoboken, NJ: John Wiley & Sons, Inc.

Szigethy, E. M. & Ruiz, P. (2001). Depression among pregnant adolescents, *American. Journal of Psychiatry,* 158 (1), 22-27, 337.

The Common Wealth Fund. (2002). Minority Americans Lag Behind Whites On Nearly Every Measure Of Health Care Quality, Retrieved from September 18, 2008 from **www.cmwf.org/newsroom/newsroom show. htm?doc id=223608** - 36k -

Tillman, L. C. (2002). Culturally sensitive Research approaches: An African American perspective. *Educational Researcher,* 31 (9) 3-11.

Tinsley-Jones, H. (2003). Racism: Calling a spade a spade. *Psychotherapy: Theory, Research, Practice, Training, 40,* 179-186.

U.S. Department of Health and Human Services (2001). *Mental health Culture, race, and ethnicity- A supplement to Mental health: A report of the Surgeon. General (DHHS* Publication No SMA 01-3613*)* Washington, DC: U.S. Government Printing Office.

Warren, B. J. (1995). Examining depression among African American Women using womanist and psychiatric mental health nursing Perspectives. *Journal of Women Theory and Research,* women@www.uga.edu.

Weinberg, M. K. Posener, J.A., DeBattista, C. Kalehzan, B.M. Rothschild, A.J. & Shear, P.K. (2001). Subsyndromal depression symptoms and major depression in postpartum women. American Journal of Orthopsychiatry, 7 (1), 87-97.

Williams, D.R., González, H.M., Neighbors, H., Nesse, R., Abelson, J.M., Sweetman, J., et al. (2007). Prevalence and distribution of Major Depressive Disorder in African Americans, Caribbean Blacks and Non Hispanic Whites: Results from the National Survey of American Life. *Archives of General Psychiatry*, 33 (4), 412-429.

Willis, L.A., Coombs, D.W., Drentea, P., & Cockerham, W.C. (2003). Uncovering the mystery: factors of African suicide. *Suicide and life-Threatening Behavior*, 33 (4), 412-429.

Wise, L.A., Krieger, N. Zierier, & Harlow, B.L. (2002). Lifetime socioeconomic position in relation to onset of peri-menopause. *Journal of Epidemiology & Community Heath*, 56 (11), 851-860.

Wolkowitz, O. (1999). Aniglucocorticoid treatment of depression: Double-blind ketoconazole. *Biological Psychiatry*, 45 (8) 1070-1074.

Yonder, K.A. Brown, W.A. (1996). Pharmacologic treatment for Premenstrual Dysphoric Disorder. *Psychiatric Annual*, 26, 586-589.

Young, S., Klap, R, Sherbourne, C.S., & Well, K.B. (2000). The quality of care for depressive and anxiety disorder in the United State. *Archives of General Psychiatric*, 58 (1), 55-61.

Zauszniewski, J. A., Picot, S. J., F., Debanne, S.M., Roberts, B. L. et al., (2002). Psychometric characteristics of the Depressive Cognition Scale in African American women.   *Journal of Nursing* Measurement, 10. 83-95.

Zung, W. Broadhead, E. & Roth, M. (1993). Prevalence of depressive symptoms in primary care. *Journal of Family Practitioner*, 37.

Appendix A: Resources for Depression

National Institute of Mental Health, NIH, HHS
6001 Executive Boulevard
Room 8184, MSC 96663
Bethesda, MD 20892-9663
Phone: (301) 496-9576
Internet Address: http://www.nimh.nih.gov

National Mental Health Information Center,
SAMHSA, HHS
P.O. Box 2345
Rockville, MD 20847
Phone: (800) 789-2647
Internet Address: http://www.mentalhealth.org

American Psychological Association
750 First Street NE,
Washington, DC 20002-4242
Phone: (800) 374-2721
Internet Address: http://www.apa.org

National Mental Health Association
2000 N. Beauregard Street 6th Floor
Alexandria, VA 22311
Phone: (800) 969-NMHA
Internet Address: http://www.nmha.org

Postpartum Education for Parents
p.o. Box 6154
Santa Barbara, CA 93160
Phone: (805) 564-3888
Internet Address: http://www.sbpep.org

Postpartum Support International
P.O. Box 60931
Santa Barbara, CA 93160
USA
Phone: (805) 967-7636
Internet Address: http://www.postpartum.net

American Geriatrics Society
The Empire State Building
350 Fifth Avenue, Suite 801
New York, NY 10118
Phone - 212/308-1414 Fax - 212/832-8646
Email - info@americangeriatrics.org
Internet Address:
www.americangeriatrics.org/educaion/forum/alz-care.shtml

National Institute for Complimentary and Alternative Medicine
National Institute of Health
9000 Rockville Pike
Bethesda, Maryland 20892, USA
Internet Address: nccam.nih.gov
E-mail :   info@nccam.nih.gov Contact NCCAM

National Alliance for the Mentally Ill
Colonial Place Three
2107 Wilson Blvd., Suite 300
Arlington, VA 22201-3042
Main Phone: (703) 524-9094
Fax: (703) 524-9094
Member Services (888) 999-NAMI (6264)
Internet address:www.nami.org

National Library of Medicine
8600 Rockville Pike

Bethesda, MD 20894
Internet address: <u>www.nlm.nih.gov/medlineplus/drug-information.html</u>

Appendix B: B. R. Kennedy Cultural Sensitive Depression Inventory Scale for Minority Groups

The Kennedy Depression Inventory is a self-rating 5-point Likert scale that measures depression. The scale is completed in 10 minutes. The total score provides an estimate of the degree of severity of the depressed mood. Add the raw scores.

Please make a check mark in the block to your response to each statement:

4 = Always
3 = Most of the Time
2 = Some of the Time
1 = Seldom
0 = Never

	Always 4 points	Most of the time 3 points	Some of the Time 2 points	Seldom 1 Point	Never 0 point
1. I feel sad, weary and the blues all the time.					
2. I am tired and have no energy.					

3. The sadness, blues, weary feelings, and lack of energy interfere with work and/or school and social life.					
4. I feel sad and weary related to completing tasks.					
5. I feel sad and weary related to health problems.					
6. I noticed when I am sad and weary I have more bodily aches and pain.					
7. I noticed when I am sad and weary I have an increase in appetite and tend to eat more.					
8. I feel discouraged about the future for minorities.					
9. The limited opportunities for minorities cause me to feel down or depressed.					

10. The limited opportunities for minorities cause me to feel irritable or angry.					
11. The limited opportunities for minorities decrease my interest in work and Seeking a job.					
12. I feel like I am being punished for some reason.					
13. I am disappointed in myself and the lack of accomplishments.					
14. I have thoughts of killing myself.					
15. I have thoughts of hurting others.					
16. I am tearful and cry a lot.					
17. I have no interest in social events etc.					
18. I find it hard making decisions concerning my life.					

19. I have difficulties sleeping at night.					
20. I overindulge when I am feeling depress with one of the following: eating, drinking alcohol, sex etc.					
21. I have no interest in sex.					
22. I will dress up regardless even though I feel down and depress.					
23. I will pray, attend religious services even when I feel down or depress.					
24.The racism, inequality and discrimination that I experience cause me to feel hopeless about the future.					
25.I continue to pray or be encourage even though I feel depress or sad.					

Please add the number of check marks in each block, and then multiply by the number at the top of block of likert scale 4, 3, 2 and 1.

Total Score	Levels of Depression
0-25	Normal
26-50	Mild Mood Changes
51-75	Moderate Depression
76-100	Severe Depression

Copyright BRK Healthcare Services, Inc

If you score within moderate to severe depression, you need to talk with healthcare professionals.

LaVergne, TN USA
10 December 2009
166630LV00009B/220/P